The Complete
DRCOG

OSCEs, MCQs and
Revi

D0263480

Commissioning Editor: Ellen Green
Project Development Manager: Siân Jarman
Project Manager: Nancy Arnott
Designer: Erik Bigland

The Complete
DRCOG
OSCEs, MCQs and Revision Notes

M. J. McCormack
MD FRCOG
Consultant Obstetrician and Gynaecologist
Countess of Chester NHS Trust, Chester

S. J. Duthie
MBChB (Liverpool) FRCOG DIP VENEREOLOGY (Liverpool)
Consultant Obstetrician and Gynaecologist
Victoria Hospital NHS Trust, Blackpool

M. A. Khaled
MRCOG
Consultant Obstetrician and Gynaecologist
Prince Charles Hospital NHS Trust, Merthyr-Tydfil

W.B. SAUNDERS
Edinburgh • London • New York • Philadelphia • St Louis • Sydney • Toronto • 2002

WB SAUNDERS
An imprint of Harcourt Publishers Limited

First published 2002

ISBN 0-7020-2583-6

British Library Cataloguing in Publication Data
A catalogue record for this book is available from the British Library

Library of Congress Cataloging in Publication Data
A catalog record for this book is available from the Library of Congress

Note
Medical knowledge is constantly changing. As new information becomes available, changes in treatment, procedures, equipment and the use of drugs become necessary. The authors and the publishers have taken care to ensure that the information given in this text is accurate and up to date. However, readers are strongly advised to confirm that the information, especially with regard to drug usage, complies with the latest legislation and standards of practice.

The
publisher's
policy is to use
**paper manufactured
from sustainable forests**

Printed in China

PREFACE

The examination leading to the Diploma in Obstetrics and Gynaecology of the Royal College for Obstetricians and Gynaecologists has changed significantly over the last few years. Recent changes in medical practice, advances in the specialty and the increased expectation from patients in terms of the information that is provided to them and the success of treatment have all altered the practice of obstetrics and gynaecology. The modern general practitioner not only requires a sound basic knowledge, clinical skills and professionalism but the 'all round' qualities of being able to communicate, counsel and audit are essential. The new style DRCOG examination, with its emphasis on objective structured clinical examination, aims to test the various qualities which the general practitioner would need from the perspective of obstetrics and gynaecology.

The purpose of this book is to address the educational needs of candidates preparing for the DRCOG examination. The book provides lecture notes and examples of the sort of questions that a candidate would have to tackle in the examination.

We, the authors, hope that you enjoy reading the book as much as we have enjoyed writing it.

September 2001

M.J.M.
S.J.D.
M.A.K.

ACKNOWLEDGEMENTS

The authors would like to acknowledge Dr R. Roberts Consultant
Paediatrician, Blackpool Victoria Hospital NHS Trust for writing
the 'Notes on neonatal paediatrics'. We also gratefully acknowledge
Dr C. O' Mahoney, Consultant in Genito-Urinary Medicine,
Countess of Chester Hospital NHS Trust, and Dr N. Murphy,
Consultant Paediatrician, Countess of Chester Hospital NHS Trust,
for their help, in preparation of the OSCE questions in
genitourinary medicine and neonatology. We thank Brenda
Middleton, secretary to Mr S.J. Duthie for her untiring assistance in
the typing of the manuscript.

CONTENTS

INTRODUCTION

1

The DRCOG examination has both formative and summative assessment and consists of three parts:

1. A 22-station Objective Structured Clinical Examination (OSCE) lasting 2 hours and 12 minutes;
2. A Multiple Choice Question (MCQ) Paper containing 60 five-part questions lasting 2 hours;
3. Satisfactory completion of six months' practical experience in obstetrics and gynaecology in a unit accredited for training; candidates successful in the examination are required to provide certified evidence of completion of training at the time of registration as a Diplomate.

Formative assessment is undertaken during the 6 months of obstetrics and gynaecology at a unit accredited for training. Trainees are assessed using a structured logbook of training completed by themselves and continual review between the trainer and trainee allows feedback and development.

This book hopes to provide adequate preparation enabling trainees to undertake the OSCE and MCQ papers successfully. It is unique in providing practice OSCE and MCQ papers in addition to comprehensive revision notes on essential topics of the syllabus for the DRCOG. To allow appropriate study and preparation, it is important to remember that the syllabus includes obstetrics, gynaecology, neonatal medicine, genitourinary medicine and contraception. Candidates should be familiar with the syllabus and regulations relating to taking the DRCOG examination and these are outlined in the booklet *Diploma Examination Regulations* which may be obtained from the Royal College of Obstetricians and Gynaecologists.

The OSCE and MCQ papers are held on the same day and candidates sit one of the examinations in the morning and the other in the afternoon. Lunch and refreshments are provided and candidates from the OSCE and MCQ components are separately confined to prevent communication before the afternoon examinations. The pass mark for the MCQ paper is 70% and for the OSCE 65%, and candidates must succeed in both components to pass the examination. Candidates should attempt all MCQs and OSCE questions as there is no negative marking. OSCE and MCQ instructions for candidates are provided from the Royal College of Obstetricians and Gynaecologists and all candidates should read these carefully. Important instructions are highlighted later in the OSCE and MCQ sections and in both there are notes relating to each question, in addition to the correct answers, which should emphasize important aspects of a particular syllabus topic.

In the DRCOG examination the time allocated for the MCQ paper is 2 hours allowing approximately 2 minutes per question with five items. The time for the OSCE is 2 hours and 12 minutes allowing 6 minutes for each of the 22 stations. It is important during your study to allocate an equivalent amount of time for a set number of questions in order to simulate examination conditions when using this book (for example 10 MCQs in 20 minutes or five OSCE questions in 30 minutes). After completing these 'tests' the answers can then be reviewed with appropriate further reading and revision undertaken as required. The OSCE has 22 stations of which 15 are factual stations, five are interactive and two are 'rest' stations. These rest stations have no questions but may provide information to prepare for the question at the next station. Appropriate types of factual question are included in the OSCE chapter with examples of interactive questions and some guidance on how these stations are best managed. It may be appropriate to supplement your preparation for the examination by attending a DRCOG course that will allow practical experience in interactive stations in addition to MCQ and OSCE questions. The RCOG can be contacted for a list of recognized courses.

This book has been designed to help your preparation for the DRCOG and we wish you every success in the examination.

THE OSCE

2

The OCSE consists of 22 stations including 15 factual or problem-solving, five interactive and two rest stations. These stations are actually desks which are arranged in a circuit of 22; there may be several circuits within the examination hall. Each candidate is informed in advance of the circuit and station number where he/she will start and a bell is sounded at 6-minute intervals allowing rotation through all stations. An answer pack is provided for each candidate with the appropriate name, candidate number and station number, and each answer sheet is collected at the end of a station. *Be careful not to mix up answer sheets as the wrong answer sheet for a question will obviously provide the wrong questions at a particular station.* The five interactive stations are located together and therefore the candidate will undertake these questions consecutively. The interactive stations are usually individually located in a room or partially separated with sound proof screens to reduce noise and distraction to other candidates.

This chapter contains 20 OSCE questions that provide typical examples of the factual questions you will encounter in the DRCOG. In the examination itself, it is important to write answers in the boxes provided as no marks are given for answers written outside a box. We have provided similar boxes in the OSCE questions on the following pages. Remember as you work through this chapter to simulate examination conditions and allow yourself the appropriate time to complete questions before referring to the answers.

INTERACTIVE STATIONS

Interactive stations are either a 'structured oral' station, or a station involving a 'surrogate patient'. Interactive stations with surrogate patients are designed to test communication skills in addition to knowledge and it is important to demonstrate satisfactory communication skills at all these stations as it is not possible to identify which stations are specifically assessing communication. It is obviously difficult to create an 'actual consultation' environment for the surrogate patient interactive stations, but it is important to remember that the examiners recognize the limitations of the situation and the candidate should try and demonstrate satisfactory communication skills during the 6-minute station.

The candidate should introduce him or herself to the patient, establish a rapport, and avoid the use of medical jargon, such as amniocentesis, karyotyping, chromosomes, salpingectomy and so on. If it is necessary to use such terms then they must be appropriately explained to the patient. Candidates must recognize both verbal and non-verbal cues which will be purposely provided by the surrogate patient during the consultation. Verbal cues are easily recognized and as an example the patient might say 'I am worried', 'I am upset' or 'I am shocked' which should then prompt an appropriate response from the candidate. Non-verbal cues are provided by the patient's facial expression or body language indicating worry, sadness, aggression or surprise as examples. All interactive stations have an examiner present to assess the candidate, and surrogate patients are also involved in allocating marks.

Many clinical scenarios are ideal for interactive surrogate patient stations and examples might include counselling a patient in the use of the oral contraceptive pill (OCP), a patient with a positive Down's serum screening result, a patient who has requested HRT or a patient who has requested emergency contraception. At each station information is usually provided to the candidate about the clinical problem. The examiner will allow you time to read this and prepare yourself before asking you to proceed with the 'consultation'.

The structured orals are essentially an oral examination on a particular clinical problem but there is a rigid structure to the questions and marking scheme, ensuring all candidates are equally assessed.

It is useful to practise interactive stations, either on a DRCOG course or by role-playing in your own unit, and four examples of questions with appropriate examiner mark sheets are shown below.

	Marks
SURROGATE PATIENT STATION QUESTION 1	

INTERACTIVE STATION EXAMPLES

You are a GP and a 16-year-old girl attends your surgery asking to start the (contraceptive) 'pill'. Counsel her appropriately.

Answer mark sheet

Examiner

1. Put patient at ease
2. Appropriate explanation of condition
3. Recognized verbal cues
4. Recognized non-verbal cues

} 8

Surrogate patient

5. Introduced him/herself to patient
6. Avoided medical jargon
7. Made appropriate eye contact
8. Listened appropriately
9. Confidence in candidate

} 1

10. Would see doctor again

1

You are an SHO in the gynaecology clinic and a 31-year-old patient is referred with a request for sterilization. She is divorced and has two children. Counsel her appropriately.

Answer mark sheet

Examiner
1. Recognized verbal/non-verbal cues
2. Counsel re: sterilization   Current contraception/partner
                                         Permanent procedure
                                         Failure rate 1–3/500
                                         Method
3. Reinforced important points

                                                                8

Surrogate patient
4. Introduced him/herself to patient
5. Avoided medical jargon   1
6. Satisfactory consultation
7. Would see doctor again   1

STRUCTURED ORAL QUESTION 1

A 21-year-old patient had a routine cervical smear which is reported as 'Moderate dyskaryosis present'. Discuss management with the examiner.

Examiner

1. What does dyskaryosis mean?
2. What is the difference between dyskaryosis and cervical intraepithelial neoplasia (CIN)?
3. How should this patient be managed?
4. What might be seen on colposcopy?
5. What treatment if any should be undertaken?
6. List three complications of treatment.
7. What is the success rate of treatment?
8. What is appropriate follow-up?

Answer mark sheet

1. Understands abnormal cell with increased nuclear/cytoplasmic ratio.   1
2. CIN is a histological diagnosis.   1
3. Needs referral for colposcopy/no further cytology follow-up.   1
4. Aceto-white lesions/punctation/mosaic areas/vessels.   1
5. Local excision transformation zone if entire lesion defined/not invasive.   2
6. Infection/haemorrhage/cervical stenosis or incompetence/recurrence.   2
7. Approximately 90%.   1
8. Colposcopy/smear 6 months; smear yearly for 5 years.   1

A 30-year-old patient is 16 weeks' gestation into her second pregnancy and has been recalled to the antenatal clinic because her maternal serum AFP result has been reported as 3.5 MOM. Discuss the counselling and management of this patient with the examiner.

Examiner
1. What is AFP?
2. Where is it produced?
3. What is the significance of this patient's result?
4. What causes do you know to account for this result?
5. How should this result be investigated?
6. If investigations confirm the fetus to have no obvious abnormality is there any risk to the continuing pregnancy?

Answer mark sheet

	Marks
1. Alpha fetoprotein.	1
2. In the yolk sac and fetal liver.	1
3. Elevated result. Normal range less than 2.5 MOM.	1
4. Causes include Wrong dates	1
Multiple pregnancy	1
Fetomaternal haemorrhage	1
Fetal abnormality (neural tube defect/abdominal wall defects)	1
5. Detailed fetal ultrasound examination.	1
6. Increased risk of IUGR, abruption, pre-eclampsia, intrauterine death. Requires increased surveillance with BP and growth monitoring.	2

A 30-year-old woman presents to the delivery suite at 33 weeks' gestation with a history of vaginal bleeding.

1. Give the definition of this complication of pregnancy.　　　2

2. List three possible causes for her bleeding.　　　3

3. List three clinical features you would look for on abdominal examination.　　　3

4. List two investigations to help confirm the diagnosis.　　　2

1. Any bleeding from the genital tract after 24 weeks' gestation until completion of the second stage of labour.
2. Local cause (cervical polyp, ectropion, infection)
   Placenta praevia
   Placental abruption
   Unexplained antepartum haemorrhage
   Vasa praevia
3. Uterine tenderness
   Abnormal lie
   High presenting part
   Fetal heart present
   Appropriate or increased uterine size
4. Ultrasound examination uterus for placental localization
   Kleihauer test for fetomaternal haemorrhage.

Comment

This patient has had an antepartum haemorrhage which is correctly defined above. Clinical assessment is very important to establish the cause of bleeding which might be from the lower genital tract or from an intrauterine cause. Placental abruption and placenta praevia are the important obstetric causes but commonly antepartum haemorrhage is unexplained. Rarely, fetal vessels crossing in the membranes of the lower uterine segment (vasa praevia) can cause antepartum haemorrhage. Clinical examination of the abdomen should confirm the presence of a normal fetal heart. Uterine tenderness, increased tone or increased uterine size might suggest an abruption and an abnormal lie or high presenting part would suggest a placenta praevia. A speculum examination is important to exclude a local cause in the genital tract. Ultrasound examination of the placenta will confirm a placenta praevia (placenta inserted in lower uterine segment) and a Kleihauer test is a blood test to identify fetal cells in the maternal circulation suggesting a placental abruption.

A 26-year-old primigravida attends the community antenatal clinic. She feels unwell. Her blood pressure is 140/85 and urinalysis confirms ++ proteinuria. Her booking blood pressure was 110/60 and urinalysis was normal.

1. List three symptoms you would ask about.   **3**

2. List three clinical signs you would look for on general examination (other than hypertension).   **3**

3. List four maternal investigations that you would arrange.   **2**

4. You assess fetal wellbeing. List two clinical signs you might find on examination of the uterus.   **2**

1. Frontal headache
   Visual disturbance
   Epigastric pain
   Nausea/vomiting
   Swelling
2. Generalized oedema
   Epigastric tenderness
   Hyper-reflexia
   Clonus
   Papilloedema
3. Full blood picture/platelet count
   Uric acid, urea and creatinine
   Liver transaminases
   24 h quantitative protein collection
4. Oligohydramnios
   Reduced fundal height

Comment

This patient has pre-eclampsia by definition, as she presents with a diastolic blood pressure more than 15 mmHg above her booking blood pressure together with proteinuria. It is important to remember the cardinal symptoms of worsening pre-eclampsia including unremitting frontal headache unrelieved by simple analgesia, visual disturbance with flashing lights or spots, and epigastric pain with nausea and vomiting. Pre-eclampsia is a multisystem disorder and thorough clincal and biochemical assessment is necessary to monitor all affected systems. Clinical examination should confirm hypertension, hyper-reflexia with clonus, epigastric tenderness and generalized oedema (pre-tibial, fingers, face, periorbital, pre-sacral, and rarely retinal). Examination of the uterus will provide evidence of IUGR and fetal compromise with reduced fundal height and oligohydramnios. Maternal blood tests are needed to investigate renal, liver and coagulation function.

A 34-year-old multiparous patient has undergone an instrumental delivery for failure to progress during the second stage of labour. You are called to the delivery suite 10 minutes following delivery because of heavy vaginal bleeding. The placenta was apparently complete.

1. What is the definition of primary post-partum haemorrhage?

   1

   delivery

2. List three causes of primary post-partum haemorrhage.

   3

3. List two clinical signs you would look for on general examination.

   2

4. List two clinical features you would confirm on pelvic examination.

   2

5. How would you manage this patient now? List two important actions.

   2

1. Bleeding from genital tract in excess of 500 ml within 24 hours of delivery
2. Uterine atony
   Retained products of conception
   Trauma to genital tract
3. Hypotension
   Pallor
   Tachycardia
   Sweating
4. Uterus well contracted
   Presence of lower genital tract trauma (vaginal/cervical tears)
   Extended episiotomy
5. Insert intravenous line and commence fluid replacement
   Check HB and crossmatch blood
   Stimulate a uterine contraction by 'rubbing' the uterus on abdominal examination
   Commence oxytocics

Comment

This patient has had a primary post-partum haemorrhage which is correctly defined above. Maternal examination will assess the extent of blood loss and the likely cause. The mother may be pale, hypotensive and sweaty, with a tachycardia indicating the need for resuscitation with fluids and blood. The only causes of post-partum haemorrhage are uterine atony, genital tract trauma and retained products. Uterine atony is the commonest cause and pelvic examination should confirm the uterus is well contracted. Immediate management with uterine atony would include 'rubbing up' a contraction. Careful inspection of the lower genital tract is needed to exclude tears of the vagina or cervix, or extension of an episiotomy which obviously needs to be sutured to achieve haemostasis. Uterine atony is managed with Syntocinon 10 IU i.v. or ergometrine 500 mg i.m. followed by an i.v. Syntocinon infusion. Vaginal or intramuscular prostaglandin is also effective. Continued maternal assessment is necessary and an examination under anaesthesia should be performed if necessary to exclude retained products of conception and trauma in the upper genital tract.

A 26-year-old primigravida is in spontaneous labour with a cephalic presentation. You are the SHO on delivery suite and are called by her midwife to reassess the patient in view of the partogram shown below.

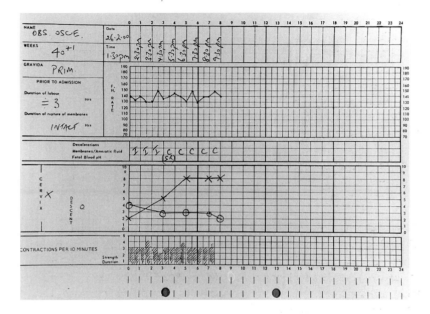

Fig. 2.1

1. What does this partogram show?

1

2. List three possible problems in labour which may cause this
   type of partogram.

3

3. You perform a pelvic examination. List four features of your
   clinical assessment.

4

4. You confirm a vertex presentation and the CTG is normal. List
   two aspects of your further management.

2

1. Secondary arrest
2. Inefficient uterine action
   Abnormal fetal position
   Cephalopelvic disproportion
3. Cervical dilatation
   Station of the head
   Position of the head
   Caput/moulding
   Liquor
   Assessment of the maternal pelvis
4. Accelerate labour with i.v. Syntocinon infusion
   Ensure adequate maternal analgesia

Comment

This is a case of a primigravida with secondary arrest. This is defined where the rate of cervical dilatation slows or stops after normal cervical progress in the active phase of labour. The three reasons for failure to progress in labour are poor uterine contractions (referred to as inefficient uterine action or dysfunctional labour), an abnormal fetal position (commonly OP position) and relative cephalopelvic disproportion indicating some disparity between the size of the fetus compared with the maternal pelvis. A careful examination is required which should include the presence of a palpable bladder, the amount of the head palpable, the cervical dilatation, position and station of the presenting part, the presence of caput and moulding and an assessment of the maternal pelvis and liquor. Other aspects include a review of the partogram and assessment of fetal and maternal wellbeing, including adequate analgesia. With normal fetal wellbeing the management would be acceleration of labour with i.v. Syntocinon and continued monitoring of the progress of labour.

A 30-year-old primigravida is 16 weeks' gestation and attends the antenatal clinic for counselling because her Down's triple serum screen test is positive with a result of 1/125.

1. What is the likely sensitivity of this test in this patient?

1

2. List three components currently used in antenatal serum screen tests.

3

3. List four important aspects of counselling.

4

4. Give two other antenatal tests which screen for chromosomal abnormalities.

2

OBSTETRIC OSCE 5 ANSWER

1. Approximately 60%
2. Total or free beta HCG
   AFP (alpha fetoprotein)
   Estriol
   PAPP-A (pregnancy-associated plasma protein A)
3. Confirm that the patient understands that the screening test is not a diagnostic test for Down's syndrome.
   Confirm the patient understands the meaning of a baby with Down's syndrome. Explain that the result indicates that the chance of a Down's syndrome baby is 1 in 125 for this pregnancy.
   Explain that further testing by amniocentesis is available to confirm the fetal karyotype.
   Explain the procedure for amniocentesis.
   Explain the associated fetal loss rate following amniocentesis is approximately 1% (1 in 100).
4. Nuchal fold translucency scanning first trimester
   Combined serum and nuchal fold translucency screening
   Ultrasound soft markers in second trimester.

Comment

Antenatal screening for chromosomal abnormalities is offered as a standard part of antenatal care. Methods of screening include the measurement of nuchal fold translucency between 10 and 13 weeks' gestation, using a serum test between 13 and 18 weeks' gestation, or a combination of both between 10 and 13 weeks' gestation. All screening tests are reported as a numerical risk and 1 in 250 is usually considered a screen 'positive' result. The commonest serum markers are AFP, total or free beta HCG, estriol, pregnancy-associated plasma protein-A and inhibin. Detection rates vary with maternal age and the particular test but serum screening would have a sensitivity between approximately 55% at the age of 30 years rising to 80% at the age of 40 years. Important aspects of antenatal counselling are listed above and patients need to be given the appropriate information both before and after screening tests.

A 24-year-old patient has been referred because of a cervical smear reporting moderately dyskaryotic cells. She attended for a colposcopy and the findings are shown in Fig. 2.2.

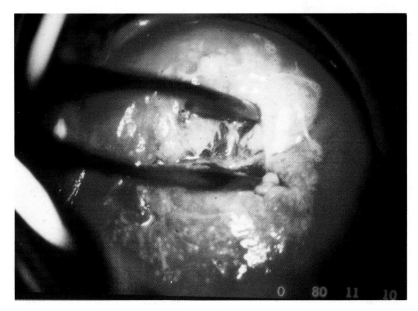

Fig. 2.2

1. Define dyskaryosis. 1

2. What abnormality is shown in Fig. 2.2 1

3. List two aspects of further management. 2

4. This patient has a large loop excision of the transformation zone. What is likely to be found at histological examination? 1

5. List three complications of this treatment. 3

6. Give an approximate success rate for this treatment. 1

7. What should be the appropriate follow up? 1

1. Abnormal-looking cells
2. Aceto-white lesion
3. Colposcopic biopsy
   Local treatment
4. CIN
5. Haemorrhage (both primary and secondary)
   Infection
   Cervical stenosis/incompetence
6. 90% success
7. Follow-up smear yearly for 5 years.

Comment
This patient was referred with a moderately dyskaryotic smear. This requires investigation by colposcopy which allows local treatment if the entire transformation zone is visualized and an invasive lesion is excluded. Aceto-white lesions are the typical colposcopic appearance of CIN. Local destructive treatments include cold coagulation, cautery, cryocautery or loop excision and all depend on complete removal or destruction of the transformation zone. Success rates following treatment are all similar and are approximately 90%. Follow-up is essential; annual cervical smears would usually be performed for 5 years before returning to routine 3-yearly recall.

A 55-year-old presents with two episodes of intermenstrual bleeding. The patient had been commenced on HRT 3 years previously for acute menopausal symptoms. Her periods were regular prior to HRT.

1. List four causes for her bleeding other than her HRT.   **4**

2. You perform a pelvic examination. List three aspects of this examination.   **3**

3. What investigations are appropriate? Name two.   **2**

4. Write a repeat prescription for her HRT.

1. Benign lower genital tract lesion (atrophic vaginitis, cervical polyp/ectropion)
   Benign endometrial cause (polyp, hyperplasia)
   Endometrial malignancy
   Cervical malignancy
   Ovarian tumour
2. Speculum assessment cervix/vagina
   Assessment of the uterus
   Assessment of the adnexa
3. Ultrasound examination of the pelvis
   Outpatient endometrial sampling
   Hysteroscopy
4. Combined cyclical oral HRT (Climagest, Nuvelle)
   Combined sequential transdermal HRT
   Transdermal oestrogen RT with cyclical oral progestogen

Comment

This patient was referred with abnormal bleeding on HRT and this requires appropriate investigation as for any patient with post-menopausal bleeding; the causes are listed above. Careful clinical examination should exclude a lower genital tract lesion but further assessment of the endometrial cavity and pelvis is needed with pelvic ultrasound and endometrial sampling. Examination under anaesthesia with hysteroscopy and endometrial curettage is a commonly performed alternative. The patient requires endometrial protection with a progestogen and would have been unsuitable for continuous combined preparations because she was still menstruating. A combined sequential preparation is needed but it may be taken either as an oral or transdermal preparation.

A woman with a regular 35-day cycle has been asked to keep a basal body temperature (BBT) chart as part of her initial infertility investigations. The hormone profile taken on day 4 of her cycle is shown below.

Normal range			
FSH	9	IU/l	(1.3–6.3)
LH	38	IU/l	(5–25)
Prolactin	200	mU/l	(< 500)
Oestrogen	100	pmol/l	(70–800)

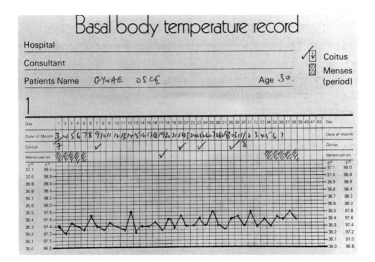

Fig. 2.3

1. What instruction would you give regarding the use of a
    BBT chart?   1

2. What does the chart provided (Fig. 2.3) show?   1

3. What is the most likely cause in this patient?   1

4. What test might help to confirm this diagnosis?   1

5. Prescribe the common medical treatment for this condition.   1

6. List two complications of this treatment.   2

7. What is the second-line medical treatment required if your
    treatment is unsuccessful?   1

8. List two methods of monitoring the treatment.   2

1. Record temperature at same time every day
2. Chart shows monophasic or anovulatory pattern
3. Polycystic ovarian syndrome (PCOS)
4. Pelvic ultrasound
5. Prescription for clomifene: clomifene 50 mg daily from days 1 to 5 of menstrual cycle for three cycles. Total 15 tabs.
6. Hyperstimulation
   Multiple pregnancy
   Hot flushes
   Dyspareunia
7. Gonadotrophin therapy
8. Oestrogen levels/ultrasound monitoring of ovarian follicles

Comment

This patient has anovulatory infertilty secondary to polycystic ovarian syndrome (PCOS). Her BBT shows a monophasic pattern and her LH:FSH ratio is greater than 3:1 consistent with the diagnosis. Ultrasound may exhibit the classical 'pearl necklace' appearance with multiple peripheral small follicles (>10) and an increased stroma. Clomifene would be the initial treatment, followed by laparoscopic ovarian diathermy. If this was unsuccessful induction of ovulation with gonadotrophin therapy would be needed. Monitoring the growth of ovarian follicles using pelvic ultrasound or urinary oestrogen levels is essential.

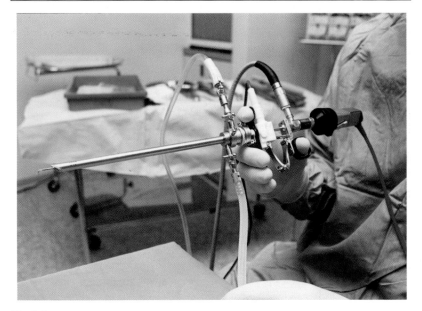

Fig. 2.4

1. What instrument is shown in Fig. 2.4? **1**

2. List two operations for which this instrument might be used. **2**

3. List three aspects of pre-operative counselling. **3**

4. List four possible complications of surgery. **4**

1. Gynaecological resectoscope
2. Resection of the endometrium
   Removal of intrauterine polyps/fibroids
3. Admission details /length of stay/advice regarding recovery and return to employment
   Brief explanation of procedure
   Common complications
   Rare need for hysterectomy (1%) and need for blood transfusion
   Pre-operative preparation of the endometrium/post-operative antibiotics
4. Primary/secondary haemorrhage
   Infection
   Uterine perforation
   Injury to bowel or bladder

Comment

Fig. 2.4 picture shows a gynaecological resectoscope used for endometrial resections and the removal of intrauterine polyps. Counselling is an important aspect of all surgery. It is important to advise regarding admission, length of stay, recovery and return to work. It is necessary to explain the procedure in simple terms so that the patient understands what is involved, and to advise about common complications and the need for likely interventions such as blood transfusion or hysterectomy. The patient needs to be informed about the need for any medication including preparations to induce endometrial atrophy prior to surgery and antibiotic prophylaxis.

A 50-year-old patient attends for investigation of urinary incontinence and the findings are shown in Fig. 2.5.

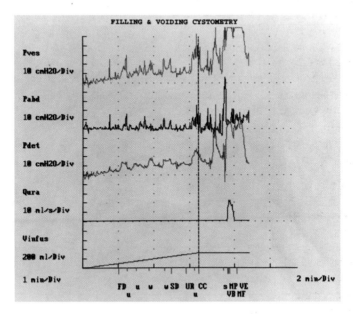

Fig. 2.5

Marks

1. List three features you would look for on pelvic examination. | 3

2. List three tests you might arrange in addition to urodynamics. | 3

3. What does the urodynamic study in Fig. 2.5 show? | 2

4. List two appropriate treatments. | 2

1. Demonstrate incontinence on coughing
   Check for uterovaginal prolapse
   Check for pelvic mass
   Confirm atrophic changes in the lower genital tract
2. Mid-stream urine culture (MSU)
   Fluid balance record chart
   Urinary flow studies
   Pad test
3. Filling cystometry/detrusor instability
4. Bladder training
   Medical therapy (oxybutynin/tolterodine)
   Oestrogen treatment
   Weight loss by dieting
   Advice relating to fluid intake

Comment

This patient was referred with urinary incontinence. This is usually stress incontinence, detrusor instability or a mixture of both. Abdominal examination will confirm whether the patient is overweight and exclude the presence of any pelvic mass or suprapubic tenderness. Pelvic examination will confirm the extent of any uterovaginal prolapse, exclude evidence of oestrogen deficiency and may demonstrate urinary incontinence on coughing. Investigations include a urinary fluid intake record to establish the nature of symptoms and to confirm normal fluid intake, MSU to exclude infection and a pad test to indicate stress incontinence. Urodynamic studies will include a urinary flow test to exclude urethral flow problems and cystometry to assess bladder function. The cystometry test studies detrusor pressure (contractions) in response to bladder filling. In normal women the maximum bladder capacity during cystometry is 500 ml and the presence of detrusor contractions greater than 15 cm H_2O during filling indicates an unstable bladder. During cystometry intravesical (Pves in Fig. 2.5) and intra-abdominal (Pabd in Fig. 2.5) pressures are recorded by placement of pressure catheters in the bladder and rectum, and subtraction of these pressures provides the detrusor pressure alone (Pdet). This report shows a slightly reduced bladder capacity and many detrusor contractions during filling confirming the diagnosis of detrusor instability (unstable bladder). Treatment is non-surgical and includes general advice about weight loss and fluid intake, bladder training and anti-cholinergic medication if necessary.

A 17-year-old patient presents to your morning surgery requesting post-coital contraception. She had unprotected intercourse the previous evening.

1. You decide to prescribe PC4. What does this contain? **1**

2. How long after intercourse may PC4 be prescribed? **1**

3. What other method of post-coital contraception is available? **1**

4. How long after intercourse may this method be used? **1**

5. List three side effects of PC4 contraception. **3**

6. List three aspects of counselling you would give this patient. **3**

1. Norgestrel 500 μg
   Ethinylestradiol 50 μg
2. First dose to be taken within 72 h of intercourse
3. IUCD
4. Within 5 days of intercourse (or up to 5 days after presumed ovulation)
5. Nausea
   Vomiting
   Headaches
   Breast tenderness
   Irregular bleeding
6. Advise on taking medication
   Side effects
   If vomiting requires further dose
   Fetal risks if unsuccessful
   Adequate follow-up
   Future contraception

Comment

This case is about emergency contraception which can be provided by use of hormonal preparations or the insertion of an IUCD. The IUCD is thought to be more effective (99–100%) compared with the combined hormonal treatment (97%).

1. List the following methods of contraception from 1 to 5 in order
   of efficacy (1 = most effective).   **2**

                    Female sterilization
                    Combined pill (< 50 µg oestrogen)
                    Mirena IUS
                    Depo-Provera
                    Progestogen-only pill

2. List five important aspects of counselling prior to female
   sterilization.   **5**

3. List three immediate complications of laparoscopic sterilization
   procedures.   **3**

1.

Method	Failure rate/100 woman years	Order
Mirena IUS	0.1–0.2	1
Female sterilization	0–0.5	2
Combined pill (< 50 µg oestrogen)	0.2–0.3	3
Depo-Provera	0–1	4
Progestogen-only pill	0.4–4	5

2. Explain method
   Failure rate
   Irreversibility
   Consider vasectomy as alternative
   Current contraception
   Side effects/complications
   Risk of ectopic pregnancy
3. Haemorrhage/abdominal wall vessel injury
   Extraperitoneal pneumoperitoneum
   Viscus injury (bowel/bladder)
   Trauma to Fallopian tubes
   Infection

Comment

This question concerns sterilization and relative contraceptive efficacy. Adequate counselling is essential prior to making a decision about permanent contraception. It is appropriate to review current contraceptive needs and past use. Explore the reasons for choosing female sterilization and if possible involve both partners. It might be better to consider male sterilization if there are obvious female medical problems increasing the risks of surgery. It should be emphasized that the procedure is permanent and irreversible but there is an accepted risk of failure of approximately 1/200. The technique of sterilization should be explained briefly and relevant complications related to which surgical technique is being performed.

A 35-year-old patient with two children aged 3 and 5 years, requests a Mirena IUS for contraception. She has a regular menstrual cycle and pelvic examination is normal.

1. Describe this device.

1

2. When should the device be inserted?

1

3. What is the contraceptive mode of action of this device?

3

4. List four side effects of this device.

4

5. Quote an efficacy rate for this device.

1

1. T-shaped silastic device with a cylindrical reservoir of levonorgestrel (52 mg) releasing 20 µg every 24 h.
2. In the first 7 days of cycle
3. Causes inflammatory reaction in genital tract impeding sperm transport and fertilization
   Alters cervical mucus to impair sperm penetration/migration
   May stop ovulation
4. Irregular menstrual bleeding/amenorrhoea
   Functional ovarian cysts
   Progestogenic symptoms (breast tenderness, acne, bloatedness, depression)
   Perforation
   Expulsion
   Increased risk of ectopic pregnancy.
5. Very effective 0.1–0.2 per 100 woman years

Comment

The Mirena intrauterine system (IUS) is the only currently available progestogen-releasing device in the UK and is licensed for 5 years. It releases 20 µg levonorgestrel in 24 h from a cylindrical reservoir of 52 mg which surrounds a silastic Nova T-shaped frame. It is very effective with a failure rate of 0.1–0.2 per 100 woman years and return of fertility is rapid after removal. Its main effects are by endometrial suppression and changes to cervical mucus but it can also interfere with ovulation. In addition it will cause a genital tract inflammatory reaction like other IUCDs. It reduces menstrual blood flow and results in amenorrhoea in about 20% of users but there is a high incidence of irregular bleeding in the first 3–6 months of use. Progestogenic side effects occur infrequently and as with any continuous progestogen functional ovarian cysts may occur. The device has the same risk of expulsion and perforation as the Nova T IUCD.

1. Give the name of a combined oral contraceptive pill (OCP).   **1**

2. List the constituents and doses.   **2**

3. List four contraindications to its use.   **4**

4. List three non-contraceptive benefits of the combined OCP.   **3**

1 and 2. You should be familiar with a few preparations. Some examples are:

Microgynon oestrogen 30 µg/levonorgestrel 150 µg
Ovysmen   oestrogen 35 µg/norethisterone 1 mg
Cilest   oestrogen 35 µg/norgestimate 250 µg

3. Cardiovascular disease
   History of venous thrombosis
   Hereditary thrombophilia
   Focal/crescendo migraine
   Active liver disease
   Known or suspected breast cancer
   Ulcerative colitis or Crohn's disease
4. Regular light painless periods
   Reduction in PMT
   Reduction in benign breast disease
   Reduction in functional ovarian cysts
   Protection against endometrial cancer and epithelial ovarian cancers
   Decreased pelvic inflammatory disease

Comment

You should have a good knowledge of the oral contraception both for the examination and your clinical practice. Combined oral contraceptives are divided into monophasic, biphasic or triphasic preparations depending on whether the dose of the oestrogen and progestogen varies during the cycle. Bi-and triphasic preparations aim to provide a total lower dose of hormones. Conditions where use of the pill is contraindicated are reviewed later. Risks of infarction or embolism are increased in patients with hypertension, ischaemic heart disease, venous thromboembolism and heavy smokers. The pill protects against carcinoma of the ovary and endometrium but may be associated with cervical and breast cancer. It should be avoided with active liver disease and gallstones.

There are many beneficial effects of the pill as outlined in the contraceptive notes (see Chapter 5).

GENITOURINARY MEDICINE OSCE 1

A 28-year-old single female presented complaining of a vaginal discharge. Fig. 2.6 shows the microscopy of a Gram-stained endocervical slide.

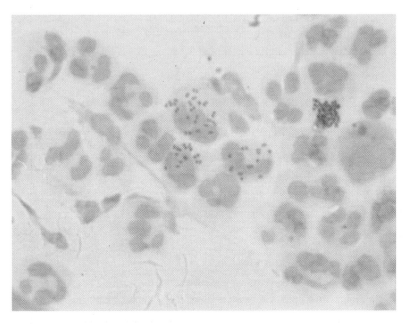

Fig. 2.6

1. Describe two features of the organism in Fig. 2.6   2

2. Name the likely organism.   1

3. Prescribe an appropriate treatment.   1

4. List three aspects of management.   3

5. List three complications.   3

1. Intracellular
   Diplococcus
   Gram-negative
2. *Neisseria gonorrhoeae*
3. Ciprofloxacin 500 mg
   Amoxicillin 2 g
   Probenicid 1 g
4. Counsel regarding the result of investigation
   Commence appropriate antibiotic
   Arrange contact tracing
   Screen for other STI
5. Pelvic inflammatory disease
   Tubo-ovarian abscess
   Infertility
   Risk of ectopic pregnancy
   Chronic pelvic pain/menorrhagia

Comment
The incidence of gonorrhoea has decreased by approximately 60% throughout the UK in the last 10 years. It is caused by *Neisseria gonorrhoeae* which is a Gram-negative intracellular diplococcus. The incubation period is usually 2 weeks and may be asymptomatic in approximately one-third of women. They may present with frequency, dysuria, cystitis, vaginal discharge, pelvic inflammatory disease or Bartholin's abscess. Gonococcal ophthalmia neonatorum may be a cause of neonatal eye infection. Treatment is usually with penicillin or a cephalosporin.

A 28-year-old married patient attends her GP complaining of a frothy vaginal discharge. The findings on examination of the external genitalia are shown in Fig. 2.7.

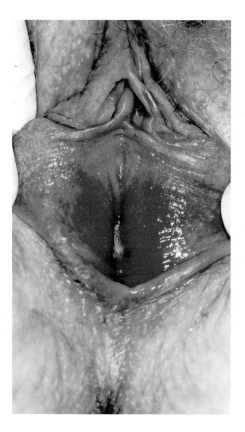

Fig. 2.7

1. Describe the characteristic feature shown in Fig. 2.7

2

[handwritten] E........... y red infection

2. What organism is likely to be responsible?

2

[handwritten] T vaginalis

3. List two tests for confirming the diagnosis.

2

[handwritten] culture

[handwritten] wet preparation

4. Describe two characteristic features of the appearance of
   this organism which allows its identification.

2

[handwritten] flagellae

5. Prescribe an appropriate treatment.

2

[handwritten] metronidazole

1. Strawberrry red appearance to introitus
2. *Trichomonas vaginalis*
3. Culture
   Wet preparation
4. Pear-shaped organism
   Flagella (four) at one end
   Undulating membrane down one side
5. Metronidazole 2 g
   Alternatively metronidazole 2–400 mg twice daily for a week

Comment

Trichomonas vaginalis is a protozoan organism which is pear-shaped, between 15 and 30 μm long. It has four flagella at its anterior end and an undulating membrane down one side. It can easily be identified on a wet film by its characteristic appearance or by culture. It causes a smelly itchy copious discharge but may be asymptomatic. With a bladder infection frequency and dysuria occur and it may be a cause of recurrent cystitis; classically it produces a strawberry-red appearance to the vulva, vagina and cervix because of inflammation and oedema. Effective treatment is with metronidazole either 2 g stat or 2–400 mg b.d. for a week.

A 26-year-old patient presents at 12 weeks' gestation. She was diagnosed as HIV positive 2 years previously and is clinically well. She has come to the antenatal clinic to discuss the implications for her pregnancy.

1. List four aspects which should be covered in your discussion. **4**

2. Give an estimate for the risk of fetal infection with HIV. **1**

3. Name two possible strategies that reduce the risk of transmission. **2**

4. What advice would you give regarding the management of labour? **3**

1. The risks of vertical transmission
   AZT prophylaxis
   Option of termination of pregnancy
   Breastfeeding
   Appropriate monitoring (viral load T4 count) and treatment for
     complications of the disease
   Management of neonate
2. 15–30% in non-breastfeeding mothers without therapeutic intervention
3. AZT treament
   Avoid breastfeeding
4. Avoid artificial rupture of membranes
   Acceleration of labour to reduce prolonged labour
   Forceps in preference to vaccum to reduce fetal trauma
   Avoid fetal blood sampling in labour
   Consideration of Caesarean section
   Staff to follow infection safe-practice guidelines

Comment

Mothers with HIV infection require careful and informed counselling
relating to the management of their pregnancy. The vertical transmission rate
appears to be about 15–30% and this can be significantly reduced with
specific measures in pregnancy. AZT treatment to the mother antenatally and
the neonate post-natally have been shown to reduce the rate. Breastfeeding
doubles the risk of HIV infection in the baby. There are some data to suggest
delivery by Caesarean section may also reduce vertical transmission.
Mothers need to be carefully monitored for complications, and joint
management with a physician experienced in the care of HIV complications
is essential. Management of labour should avoid the risk of fetal infection by
avoiding rupture of membranes, avoiding prolonged labour by appropriate
acceleration, avoiding fetal blood sampling and using forceps in preference
to vacuum to reduce skin trauma. Strict attention should be given to
procedures minimizing the risk of infection to staff.

The RCOG Working Party Report on HIV in maternity care and
gynaecology (1997) is recommended reading.

1. What are the components of the APGAR score? | 2

> *HR (handwritten)*
> *Colour*
> *Muscle tone*
> *Respiration*
> *Irritability (Reflex)*

2. Allocate the correct score for a baby with each of the following. | 3
   Heart rate below 100 bpm
   Pink body with blue extremities
   Grimacing

3. List five important aspects of resuscitation of the newborn. | 5

> *call for help*
> *neutral position*
> *dry + keep warm*

1. APGAR is scoring system for assessment of the neonate performed at 1 and 5 minutes after birth. The five components below are used to provide a maximum score of 10 with each component scoring 0–2.
   Heart rate
   Respiratory effort
   Muscle tone
   Reflex irritability
   Colour

2.

Heart rate below 100 bpm	1
Pink body with blue extremities	1
Grimacing	1

3. Note time when resuscitation started
   Call for additional help
   Dry and keep warm – cover head and use radiant heater
   Clean airway/suction
   Assess at 1 minute and commence face-mask ventilation if breathing irregular or heart rate < 100 bpm
   Consider opiate antagonist if opiates given prior to delivery
   If heart rate < 60 bpm commence chest compressions

Comment

An APGAR score is traditionally used to assess the condition of the neonate at birth and was designed as a guide for the need for resuscitation. It is recorded at 1 and 5 minutes with further recordings at 5-minute intervals if resuscitation continues. The APGAR scoring system is shown below.

Component	Score of 0	Score of 1	Score of 2
Heart rate	Absent	Below 100/min	Above 100/min
Respiratory effort	Absent	Weak	Good crying
Muscle tone	Flaccid	Flexion extremities	Well flexed
Reflex irritability	No response	Grimace	Cough or sneeze
Colour	Pale or blue	Pale/blue extremities	Completely pink

Initial assessment of the neonate should indicate if resuscitation is required and the time should be noted for subsequent interpretation. Heat loss should be minimized by drying the baby and wrapping it in a warm towel with the head covered. If resuscitation is required it should be placed under a radiant heater. The airway should be cleared and usually aspiration of the upper airway with a suction device is not required. At 1 minute the condition should be assessed and if regular respiration has not been established or the heart rate is below 100/min ventilation is required. Expert paediatric help should be called for while continuing resuscitation measures. The nares and mouth should be cleared with a suction catheter and ventilation commenced with a face mask. If the heart beat remains below 100/min ventilation should be continued until spontaneous respiration has occurred. Endotracheal intubation should be considered if there is no spontaneous respiratory effort. If the heart rate falls below 60/min chest compressions should be commenced. Ventilation should continue at 60 inflations per min with 120 chest compressions/min at a rate of 3–5 compressions per inflation. Adrenaline, bicarbonate and fluid replacement may be required if continued resuscitation is required.

A term infant is noted to be jaundiced within 24 h of birth.

1. List three likely causes. **3**

Rh / ABO   *incompatible climate*

Infection

2. List four investigations you would undertake. **4**

3. List three aspects of management. **3**

1. Haemolysis from rhesus
   Haemolysis from ABO incompatibility or red-cell defects
   Congenital infection

2. Bilirubin levels
   Full blood picture
   Coombs test
   Infection screen
   Blood gases
   Kleihauer test

3. Ensure adequate hydration
   Commence serum bilirubin action chart
   Arrange phototherapy/exchange transfusion as required
   Confirm diagnosis and manage accordingly

Comment

Jaundice occurs in 50% of neonates. In the majority it is physiological and occurs after 24 h, rises to a peak (> 220 mmol/l) on day 3–4 and resolves by day 7–10. Jaundice is non-physiological and requires investigation if it occurs less than 24 h after birth, the baby is unwell, serum bilirubin exceeds 220 mmol/l (250 mmol/l in pre-term babies) or is unresolved beyond 10 days. Causes of jaundice before 24 h are listed above and require appropriate investigation. Bilirubin is toxic to the brain (kernicterus) and will cause poor feeding, irritability, hypertonicity, apnoea and convulsions and may result in cerebral palsy, deafness or mental retardation. To avoid bilirubin toxicity serum levels are carefully monitored on bilirubin charts and action levels are indicated for commencing phototherapy or exchange transfusion.

You are the SHO who is called to see a neonate 12 hours after birth because he is fitting.

1. List four likely causes for this problem.   **4**

2. List three investigations you would arrange urgently.   **3**

3. List three aspects of immediate management.   **3**

1. Perinatal asphixia/hypoxic ischaemic encephalopathy
   Metabolic problem (hypoglycaemia, hypocalcaemia, hypernatraemia)
   Infections (meningitis, septicaemia, congenital infection)
   Inborn error of metabolism
2. Blood glucose
   Serum electrolytes, Ca, Mg
   Blood gases
   Infection screen
   Cranial ultrasound
3. Check airway, administer facial O_2
   Check BM and give i.v. glucose if low
   Anti-convulsants if still fitting
   Investigate and treat cause

Comment

Neonatal seizures occur in approximately 1% of all births and can present with subtle movements or focal/generalized tonic–clonic seizure. Likely causes are listed above and require appropriate investigation for confirmation. Initial management includes maintaining airway, ensuring oxygenation and stopping fitting with anti-convulsants. The diagnosis needs to be confirmed and appropriate treatment initiated.

THE MCQ EXAMINATION

3

HOW TO ANSWER MULTIPLE CHOICE QUESTIONS

The section on multiple choice questions is designed to test factual knowledge of the syllabus including obstetrics, gynaecology, reproductive medicine, genitourinary medicine and family planning.

There is 'no negative' marking but you have to be careful in guessing the questions you are not sure of.

Multiple choice questions will have a stem and series of five answers. You have to read the stem and make *absolutely certain* that you do understand the question. If you are not sure, read the stem and relate it to the question each time. You are then required to judge whether each answer given is true or false, and note this down.

Negative statements need careful consideration and you may not score any marks if you do not consider the negative meaning of the statement.

The first impression is usually the right answer, but this is not the case with all the questions.

Try to answer the questions which you are absolutely certain about, going through the whole paper, and then come back and read through the questions that you have left and try to have another go on them. Leave the questions you are not sure about until the end.

At the end of the day, you have to make your own judgement on the questions which you could not find any way of answering. The English language can be very difficult on occasions, and words such as 'often', 'usually', 'occasionally' and 'not infrequent' (and so on) may confuse you.

Read through the question again before you commit yourself to an answer and risk not scoring a mark. This may be the difference between pass and failure.

Remember that the examiner usually puts straightforward questions in most cases and will not be looking to deceive the candidate.

Make sure that you read the statement and try to see why this question is there, answering it accordingly. There are certain topics which you *must* cover as a general practitioner and they are of interest in obstetrics and gynaecology. The guidelines produced by the RCOG are of great importance for a good standard of practice. Try to spend some time reading through these from their Website.

Topics such as problems in pregnancy, current gynaecological problems and family planning must be covered in a satisfactory way before appearing for the examination.

Family planning is an equally important part of the syllabus and you should not forget this, not only for exam purposes, but also for your own daily practice. There will be many questions on the subject of contraception, as this is an area that general practitioners will be dealing with in their daily practice.

Make sure that you have read the instructions on how to answer these MCQs from the guidance provided by the Royal College. This will keep you up to date with any changes.

Use the correct pencil and eraser, as these questions will be corrected using a computer that is very sensitive to the changes you make when answering the questions.

In the Appendix of this book, there is a sample answer sheet for MCQs (see p. 232).

The only way of improving your performance in MCQs is to practice as many questions as possible.

MULTIPLE CHOICE QUESTIONS

1. **The following are true of birth trauma:**
   (a) Fits and irritability are the earliest sign of intracranial haemorrhage.
   (b) Cephalohaematoma is usually associated with subsequent brain damage.
   (c) Should facial palsy develop due to forceps delivery it resolves within 2–3 days.
   (d) Brachial plexus injury usually involves C3/C4/C5, causing Erb's palsy.
   (e) About 50% of pre-term babies suffer spontaneous intraventricular haemorrhage.

2. **Oestrogens have the following actions:**
   (a) Pituitary stimulation
   (b) Development of secondary sexual characteristics
   (c) Fusion of the epiphysis
   (d) Decreased cervical mucus
   (e) Prevention of thrombosis

3. **Progestogens are known to cause the following:**
   (a) Decreased body temperature
   (b) Increased cervical mucus
   (c) Pituitary inhibition
   (d) Secretory changes mainly in the uterus and the breast
   (e) They prevent the onset of labour.

4. **Regarding primary amenorrhoea:**
   (a) Failure of breast development by the age of 10 requires investigation.
   (b) Kalman's syndrome is a recognized cause.
   (c) It may be due to systemic disease.
   (d) The minority of cases of primary amenorrhoea are constitutional.
   (e) Turner's syndrome is a known cause and should be excluded.

5. **In testicular feminization syndrome:**
   (a) There are usually normal testes.
   (b) Female internal organs are usually present.
   (c) Breast development is usually lacking.
   (d) There is usually a high testosterone level.
   (e) The karyotype is XX.

6. **In Turner's syndrome the following are usually observed:**
   (a) The ovaries are usually well developed.
   (b) The nipples are widely spaced.

(c) The girl is of normal stature.

(d) Aortic stenosis is a characteristic feature.

(e) The condition can be diagnosed by chromosomal analysis.

7. **Convulsions in the neonate may be due to:**
   (a) Hyperglycaemia
   (b) Hypercalcaemia
   (c) Meningitis
   (d) Cerebral oedema
   (e) Septicaemia

8. **Severe constipation in the neonate may be due to:**
   (a) Hirschsprung's disease
   (b) Hyperthyroidism
   (c) Hypocalcaemia
   (d) Diabetes mellitus
   (e) Diabetes insipidus

9. **In a neonate hypothermia can present with the following signs:**
   (a) Weak cry
   (b) Poor sucking
   (c) Twitching
   (d) Oedema of the hands and feet
   (e) Scleroderma

10. **The following are correct regarding neonatal jaundice:**
    (a) If it occurs on day 1 it is usually physiological.
    (b) Haemolytic jaundice presents on the second or third day.
    (c) Neonatal jaundice is considered after 10 days.
    (d) Prolonged jaundice is considered after 10 days.
    (e) If the Coombs test is negative, haemolysis is due to Rh incompatibility.

11. **The following are true of breastfeeding in the neonate:**
    (a) Breast milk has less lactose when compared with cow's milk.
    (b) Breast milk has more protein when compared with cow's milk.
    (c) Breast milk has the same quantity of fat with a high level of polyunsaturated fats.
    (d) There is a possible bactericidal effect when compared with cow's milk.
    (e) The gut of breastfed babies is virtually sterile.

12. **With regard to congenital abnormalities:**
    (a) Congenital dislocation of the hip is commoner in boys.
    (b) Congenital dislocation of the hip is usually treated with a Von Rosen splint.

(c) Hydrocephalus in the neonate can usually be diagnosed by measuring the head circumference.
(d) Congenital cleft lip is repaired at about 6 months.
(e) Breastfeeding is usually contraindicated in babies with cleft lip.

13. **In relation to the intrauterine contraceptive device (IUCD) the following are true:**
    (a) The multiload has the highest rates of perforation.
    (b) It is contraindicated when breastfeeding.
    (c) It can be used as a method of post-coital contraception up to 2 weeks after intercourse.
    (d) It is not contraindicated with a history of previous ectopic pregnancy.
    (e) Previous Caesarean section is an absolute contraindication.

14. **The progesterone-only pill (POP) is contraindicated in:**
    (a) Previous ectopic pregnancy
    (b) Hypertriglyceridaemia
    (c) A breastfeeding mother
    (d) Previous ectopic pregnancy
    (e) Undiagnosed vaginal bleeding

15. **The combined oral contraceptive pill (COC), besides being used as a method of contraception, can be used to treat the following:**
    (a) Endometriosis
    (b) Ovulation pain
    (c) Menorrhagia
    (d) Dysmenorrhoea
    (e) Physiological ovarian cysts

16. **The following are known contraindications to the use of the COC:**
    (a) Deep venous thrombosis or pulmonary embolus
    (b) Active liver disease
    (c) Benign intracranial hypertension
    (d) Heavy smoking and patient age over 40
    (e) Cholestasis in pregnancy

17. **The following are true of hyperprolactinaemia:**
    (a) Taking the low-dose combined oral contraceptive pill is the commonest cause of hyperprolactinaemia.
    (b) Bromocriptine acts by reducing the actual volume of microprolactinomas by about 20–30% or more.
    (c) Breastfeeding in contraindicated in women with prolactinomas.
    (d) Bromocriptine is a well-known teratogen.
    (e) A pregnant woman with prolactinoma should continue using a dopamine agonist throughout pregnancy.

18. The following agents are used in ovulation induction in patients undergoing assisted conception:
    (a) Clomifene citrate
    (b) Human menopausal gonadotrophin
    (c) Gonadotrophin-releasing hormone analogues
    (d) Human chorionic gonadotrophin
    (e) Aspirin

19. The following are known criteria for diagnosing polycystic ovarian disease (PCO):
    (a) Decreased body weight
    (b) Hormonal evidence of androgen excess
    (c) Chronic anovulation
    (d) Recurrent miscarriage
    (e) Inappropriate gonadotrophin secretions

20. The following are true of McCune–Albright syndrome:
    (a) It includes an association of fibrous dysplasia of the skeletal system and generalized cutaneous pigmentation.
    (b) Puberty is usually delayed.
    (c) The condition affects boys more than girls.
    (d) There is an autonomous hyperfunctioning of the peripheral target glands.
    (e) Menarche in this condition may occur in infancy.

21. The following can be considered as differential diagnoses of chronic pelvic pain in adolescent girls:
    (a) Endometriosis
    (b) Dysmenorrhoea
    (c) Ovarian cyst
    (d) Pelvic congestion
    (e) Hydronephrosis

22. The following are known causes of incontinence:
    (a) Ectopic ureters
    (b) Interstitial cystitis
    (c) Stroke
    (d) Diuretics
    (e) Depression

23. The following can add to the difficulty in diagnosing pelvic inflammatory disease:
    (a) Endometriosis
    (b) Adnexal torsion
    (c) Corpus luteum bleeding

(d) Pelvic adhesions
(e) Renal colic

24. **The following are related to premature ovarian failure:**
    (a) There are decreased levels of oestrogen.
    (b) It is associated with autoimmune disease.
    (c) There are decreased levels of FSH.
    (d) It is seen in association with autoimmune disease.
    (e) Karyotype is indicated in women who develop the problem before 25 years of age.

25. **Placenta praevia is more likely to be found in a pregnancy associated with:**
    (a) Multiple pregnancy
    (b) Previous manual removal of the placenta
    (c) Pyometra
    (d) IVF pregnancy
    (e) Previous Caesarean section

26. **Urinary tract infection (UTI) in pregnancy:**
    (a) Occurs in about 10% of pregnancies.
    (b) Can easily be diagnosed when there are more than 1000 bacteria per ml on culture.
    (c) Is commoner in multigravida when compared with primigravida.
    (d) May lead to pre-term labour.
    (e) If recuring necessitates investigations after delivery.

27. **The following maternal infections may cross the placenta:**
    (a) Herpes genitalis
    (b) Parvovirus B19
    (c) Toxoplasmosis
    (d) Chicken pox
    (e) Cytomegalovirus

28. **Pulmonary embolism is commoner:**
    (a) Following a normal vaginal delivery when compared with operative delivery.
    (b) In 90% of cases, when the signs of deep-vein thrombosis will precede the condition.
    (c) If a ventilation perfusion scan is absolutely contraindicated during pregnancy.
    (d) As one of the leading causes of maternal death.
    (e) With the use of aspirin, which is an associated risk factor.

29. **In severe hyperemesis gravidarum:**
    (a) The incidence is approximately 10/1000 in the UK.
    (b) It is commoner in molar pregnancies.
    (c) Therapeutic termination of the pregnancy may be necessary.
    (d) Admission is always indicated.
    (e) The condition is likelier when the fetus is male.

30. **Spermatogenesis may be inhibited by the following drugs:**
    (a) Monoamine oxidase inhibitors
    (b) Nitrofurantoin
    (c) Anti-malarials
    (d) Sulfasalazine
    (e) Aspirin

31. **Spontaneous pre-term labour may be due to:**
    (a) Polyhydramnios
    (b) Pyelonephritis
    (c) Candida infection
    (d) Previous Caesarean section
    (e) An acute attack of gastroenteritis.

32. **The following conditions are sex-linked disorders:**
    (a) Ehlers–Danlos syndrome
    (b) Hunter mucopolysaccharidosis
    (c) Duchenne muscular dystrophy
    (d) Thalassaemia
    (e) Gestational diabetes

33. **Ectopic pregnancy may be associated with:**
    (a) In vitro fertilization and embryo transfer
    (b) Previous bowel surgery
    (c) Depo-Provera
    (d) Previous laparoscopic sterilization
    (e) Previous Caesarean section

34. **The following statements are correct:**
    (a) The cause of the majority of cases of recurrent miscarriage remains unidentified.
    (b) Recurrent miscarriage affects about 10–15% of women in the reproductive age group.
    (c) Bed-rest may help prevent recurrent miscarriage.
    (d) The chances of pregnancy after one miscarriage are less than 50%.
    (e) Recurrent miscarriage can be prevented by the use of aspirin and heparin.

35. **Urethral carbuncles:**
    (a) May lead to post-menopausal bleeding.
    (b) May lead to malignant change, so they should always be removed.
    (c) Are usually symptomatic.
    (d) Are usually granulomatous lesions.
    (e) May mimic prolapsed urethral mucosa.

36. **Uterine fibroids are:**
    (a) Commoner in those of Afro-Caribbean ethnicity.
    (b) Always symptomatic.
    (c) Possibly the main cause of infertility.
    (d) Not reducible in size by medical treatment.
    (e) Known to cause backache.

37. **Imperforate hymen is:**
    (a) Easily identified early in life.
    (b) May pass unnoticed.
    (c) A known cause of haematosalpinx.
    (d) A cause of infertility.
    (e) Commoner in certain ethnic groups.

38. **In premature ovarian failure:**
    (a) Family history may be positive.
    (b) May be due to iatrogenic causes.
    (c) Occurs in 1–5% of women.
    (d) Should always be confirmed surgically.
    (e) Infection may be the cause.

39. **Concerning outpatient endometrial sampling diagnostic procedures:**
    (a) These should always be undertaken in hospital.
    (b) A negative result rules out endometrial carcinoma.
    (c) Bed-rest for at least 24 h is advisable following the procedure.
    (d) They may be performed using a pipelle in general practice.
    (e) Tissues obtained may not be sufficient for diagnosis.

40. **Genuine stress incontinence is associated with:**
    (a) Increasing parity.
    (b) A younger age group.
    (c) Decreased intra-abdominal pressure.
    (d) The menopause.
    (e) Connective tissue disorders.

41. **The following are correct regarding trophoblastic disease:**
    (a) Complete hydatidiform moles are usually homozygous 46 XX and derived solely from the father.

(b) Women with trophoblastic disease could easily be followed up in general practice.

(c) Once diagnosed, subsequent pregnancy is contraindicated.

(d) Women with trophoblastic disease should never use the oral contraceptive pill.

(e) The incidence is commoner in certain ethnic groups.

42. **The following statements are correct:**

    (a) Anti-D antibodies arise from failure in giving prophylaxis in about 30% of cases.

    (b) In Rhesus negative mothers, antibody testing is necessary on at least two occasions.

    (c) 10% of Rhesus negative women become sensitized during their pregnancy.

    (d) Women with Rhesus negative blood group should never be followed up in the community.

    (e) Anti-D should always be given to Rh negative women, even after very early proven miscarriages.

43. **Concerning the condition of vulvodynia:**

    (a) The pain of vulval vestibulitis occurs usually in response to pressure.

    (b) Essential vulvodynia has warning signs.

    (c) Lichen sclerosis may present in younger age groups.

    (d) In vulval vestibulitis dyspareunia is a common presentation.

    (e) Steroid therapy in the community is necessary to treat cases with lichen sclerosis.

44. **Some identifiable causes of stillbirth include:**

    (a) Maternal hypertension

    (b) Isoimmunization

    (c) Infections

    (d) Cord accidents

    (e) Chromosomal abnormalities

45. **The risk factors for recurrence of pre-term labour include:**

    (a) Abruption

    (b) Placenta praevia

    (c) Previous pre-term delivery

    (d) Smoking

    (e) Chorioamnionitis

46. **The following are true of HIV virus:**

    (a) When present it has no influence of the mode of delivery.

    (b) The virus can be isolated from cervical secretions.

    (c) It is a retrovirus.

(d) True incidence varies from one community to another.

(e) Vertical transmission is unlikely to happen.

47. **The following are known complications of diabetes in pregnancy:**

   (a) Increase in the incidence of congenital abnormalities.

   (b) Development of pregnancy-induced hypertension.

   (c) Development of oligohydramnios.

   (d) Development of retinopathy.

   (e) Jaundice.

48. **The following are considered as relative contraindications to the usage of HRT:**

   (a) Moderate hypertension

   (b) Mild hypercholesterolaemia

   (c) Varicose veins

   (d) Excessive alcohol consumption

   (e) Heavy cigarette smoking

49. **The following are true of carcinoma of the cervix:**

   (a) The lesion originates within the transformation zone in the majority of cases.

   (b) The disease is more common in multiparous women.

   (c) It is unlikely to produce ureteric obstruction.

   (d) The lesion is typically squamous in nature.

   (e) Spread to the iliac nodes is usual.

50. **The following are true of congenital dislocation of the hip:**

   (a) The condition is four times more common among girls.

   (b) It is associated with breech presentation.

   (c) It is best diagnosed clinically.

   (d) Fewer than 10% of cases will require further surgical correction.

   (e) There is usually an associated congenital abnormality.

51. **The condition of placental abruption is associated with:**

   (a) External cephalic version.

   (b) Nulliparous women, among whom it is more common.

   (c) Direct trauma, which may be the main cause.

   (d) A clinical diagnosis.

   (e) Always presents with vaginal bleeding.

52. **The following are true of the condition of prolapse of the umbilical cord:**

   (a) The condition is less likely to occur with brow presentation.

   (b) It complicates 1/3000 deliveries.

   (c) The main cause of fetal distress is the spasm from cooling.

(d) It is a known cause of perinatal morbidity.

(e) It is unlikely to occur with breech presentation.

53. **Vomiting in the second trimester of pregnancy may be caused by:**
    (a) Acute kidney problems
    (b) Hydatidiform mole
    (c) Inflammatory bowel conditions
    (d) Food poisoning
    (e) Ectopic pregnancy

54. **Ovarian cancer is more likely to occur in:**
    (a) Nulliparous women.
    (b) Women who have breast cancer.
    (c) Patients with a history of prolonged use of the oral contraceptive pill.
    (d) Women with a family history of ovarian cancer.
    (e) Low socio-economic classes.

55. **The following statements apply to endometriosis:**
    (a) When mild it may lead to infertility.
    (b) It is commoner after the birth of a child.
    (c) It is always symptomatic.
    (d) Depo-Provera is a known treatment.
    (e) It is characteristically associated with the development of endometrial cancer in later life.

56. **Hysteroscopy:**
    (a) Is contraindicated during menstruation.
    (b) Must be done under general anaesthetic.
    (c) Could be used to identify an endometrial polyp.
    (d) Is contraindicated by previous pelvic inflammatory disease.
    (e) Is essential in all women with abnormal menstrual bleeding below the age of 30.

57. **Retroversion of the uterus:**
    (a) Is a normal finding in about 60% of women.
    (b) May lead to backache in pregnancy.
    (c) Is an unlikely cause of urine retention during pregnancy.
    (d) Needs treatment and correction in the majority of cases.
    (e) Is a known cause of miscarriage.

58. **Congenital abnormalities of the uterus:**
    (a) Are a known cause of infertility.
    (b) May lead to miscarriage.
    (c) Are associated with malpresentation in pregnancy.
    (d) May be associated with renal abnormalities.
    (e) May be diagnosed with hysterosalpingogram.

59. Regarding ovarian cysts in pregnancy:
 (a) The dermoid accounts for up to 50% of total.
 (b) They are commonly malignant in origin.
 (c) Corpus luteal cysts account for the majority of cases.
 (d) Torsion does not occur during pregnancy.
 (e) They rarely cause obstructive labour.

60. Continuous electronic fetal monitoring in labour is highly indicated in:
 (a) Multiple pregnancies
 (b) Breech presentations
 (c) Hypertensive mothers
 (d) Pre-term infants
 (e) Intrauterine growth retardation

61. Breech presentation:
 (a) Accounts for up to 3% of term pregnancies.
 (b) May be diagnosed on clinical examination of the abdomen.
 (c) May be associated with fetal abnormality.
 (d) Is a contraindication for vaginal delivery.
 (e) Makes intrapartum hypoxia more likely than is true of cephalic presentation.

62. The following are known causes of pre-term labour:
 (a) Maternal pyrexia
 (b) Intrauterine fetal death
 (c) Polyhydramnios
 (d) Multiple pregnancy
 (e) Cervical incompetence

63. The following are known contraindications to the usage of tocolysis in pregnancy:
 (a) Cardiac disease
 (b) Severe hypertension
 (c) Clinical chorioamnionitis
 (d) Intrauterine death
 (e) Thyroid disease

64. The following may be indicative of chorioamnionitis:
 (a) Maternal pyrexia
 (b) Maternal bradycardia
 (c) Tender uterus
 (d) Fetal bradycardia
 (e) Increased white-cell count in the mother.

65. The following are true of cleft palate:
   (a) There may be a gap in the alveolar arch.
   (b) Surgery carries the best result if performed immediately after delivery.
   (c) Surgery is best performed in the first month.
   (d) Despite corrective surgery recurrent otitis media is likely to occur.
   (e) It may be associated with hearing problems.

66. In diaphragmatic hernia:
   (a) The incidence is 1/100.
   (b) The majority of cases occur on the right side.
   (c) It is unlikely to be diagnosed antenatally.
   (d) It requires intensive care and surgery when stable.
   (e) It can present with respiratory distress at birth.

67. In Down's syndrome:
   (a) The overall incidence varies but it is usually 1/600.
   (b) The nose is usually small and there is a flared nasal bridge.
   (c) There is usually a short broad neck.
   (d) Duodenal atresia usually presents.
   (e) There is generally hypotonia.

68. In Turner's syndrome:
   (a) The incidence is 1/5000.
   (b) There is usually a short webbed neck.
   (c) There are widely spaced nipples.
   (d) Oedema of the feet is a characteristic feature.
   (e) Coarctation of the aorta is usually present.

1. **(a)** True
   (b) False
   (c) False
   (d) False
   (e) True
   Cephalohaematoma is usually noticed by day 3. This is a sub-periosteal swelling, which is limited by sutures. Very rarely it can be large and may require transfusion. There is usually no brain damage associated with cephalohaematoma.
   When developed, facial palsy resolves in 2–3 weeks; if it develops the exposed cornea must be protected with hypromellose drops. Brachial plexus injury usually involves C5/C6 causing what is known as 'waiter's tip syndrome' (Erb's palsy).

2. **(a)** False
   (b) True
   (c) True
   (d) False
   (e) False
   Oestrogens usually cause pituitary inhibition; they increase cervical mucus production and exogenous oestrogens may cause an increase in the risk of thrombosis. They are used in combined oral contraceptive pills and hormone replacement therapy after the menopause.

3. **(a)** False
   (b) False
   (c) True
   (d) True
   (e) True
   Progestogens raise the body temperature and usually decrease cervical mucus.

4. **(a)** False
   (b) True
   (c) True
   (d) False
   (e) True
   Failure of breast development by the age of 14 merits investigation. Most cases of primary amenorrhoea are usually constitutional and a family history of late puberty is frequently obtained.

5. **(a)** True
   (b) False

(c) False
(d) True
(e) False
In testicular feminization syndrome the karyotype is usually XY. There is usually good breast development and a normal phenotype, but there are no internal female organs.

6. **(a)** False
   (b) True
   (c) False
   (d) False
   (e) True
   In Turner's syndrome there is ovarian dysgenesis, the so-called streak ovaries. The girls are of short stature and coarctation of the aorta is usually present. Clinical features include a webbed neck, widely-spaced nipples, a wide carrying angle at the elbow and the metatarsals are usually short.

7. **(a)** False
   (b) False
   (c) True
   (d) True
   (e) True
   Convulsions in the neonate may be due to hypoglycaemia and hypocalcaemia.

8. **(a)** True
   (b) False
   (c) False
   (d) True
   (e) True
   Hypothyroidism and hypercalcaemia are known causes of a persistent constipation.

9. **(a)** True
   (b) True
   (c) True
   (d) True
   (e) True

10. **(a)** False
    (b) False
    (c) True
    (d) True
    (e) False

Physiological jaundice appears on the second or third day while haemolytic jaundice occurs on day 1. Haemolysis is usually due to Rh incompatibility, and is more commonly due to ABO incompatibility when, for example, the mother is often group O and the baby is blood group A (it is usually mild). Remember that Coombs-negative haemolysis usually occurs due to spherocytosis or G6PD deficiency.

11. **(a)** False
    (b) False
    (c) True
    (d) True
    (e) True
    Breast milk has more lactose and less protein when compared with cow's milk.

12. **(a)** False
    (b) True
    (c) True
    (d) False
    (e) False
    Congenital dislocation of the hip is more common in girls and after a breech delivery. In cleft lip and cleft palate the lip is usually repaired at about 3 months whereas the palate is repaired at 12 months. Breastfeeding is usually possible in babies with a cleft lip.

13. **(a)** False
    (b) False
    (c) False
    (d) False
    (e) False
    The multiload IUCD has low rates of perforation. The IUCD can be used when breastfeeding and can be used as a method of post-coital contraception within 3–5 days. Previous ectopic pregnancy is a contraindication for an IUCD but previous Caesarean section is not; however a device with a low perforation rate such as the multiload is advisable.

14. **(a)** True
    (b) True
    (c) False
    (d) True
    (e) True
    The progesterone-only pill does not suppress lactation and the hormone is excreted in minute amounts in breast milk; therefore there is no known adverse effect on the baby.

15. (a) True
(b) True
(c) True
(d) True
(e) False
It is important to note that with the use of the COC there is a decreased incidence of benign breast conditions, ectopic pregnancy, ovarian and endometrial cancer and functional ovarian cysts.

16. (a) True
(b) True
(c) True
(d) True
(e) True
Remember to study all aspects related to family planning prior to your exam.

17. (a) False
(b) True
(c) False
(d) False
(e) False
The low-dose oestrogen content of the current oral contraceptive does not usually produce hyperprolactinaemia. Breastfeeding is not contraindicated in women with prolactinomas. It is important to note that the use of the prolactin level as a tumour marker during pregnancy in women with hyperprolactinaemia is of no useful value.

It is of interest to note that there is a well-described association between hyperprolactinaemia and polycystic ovaries. The real cause for this association is not yet known. An alternative dopamine agonist for treatment is cabergoline.

18. (a) True
(b) True
(c) True
(d) True
(e) False
Aspirin is not used as an agent for ovulation induction.

19. (a) False
(b) True
(c) True
(d) True
(e) True
In PCO there is usually increased body weight rather than decreased body weight.

20. (a) False
  (b) False
  (c) False
  (d) True
  (e) True
  This syndrome is the result of an association of fibrous dysplasia of the skeletal system with patchy pigmentation and precocious pubertal development. The condition usually affects girls more than boys and there is no racial predominance.

21. (a) True
  (b) True
  (c) True
  (d) True
  (e) True
  Consider all of these when managing patients with chronic pelvic pain.

22. (a) True
  (b) True
  (c) True
  (d) True
  (e) True
  All the above, plus others, are known causes of incontinence.

23. (a) True
  (b) True
  (c) True
  (d) True
  (e) True
  Pelvic inflammatory disease can be difficult to diagnose because of the presence of any of the above. It is also difficult to diagnose in the presence of internal gastrointestinal bleeding or gastrointestinal infections, lower-lobe pneumonia, acute appendicitis and mesenteric adenitis or ischaemic bowel problems.

24. (a) True
  (b) True
  (c) False
  (d) True
  (e) True
  Premature ovarian failure is diagnosed in women before the age of 40, who usually present with symptoms of hypo-oestrogenism, an increased level of FSH and generalized sclerosis in association with autoimmune disease.

25. **(a)** True
    (b) False
    (c) False
    (d) False
    (e) True
    Placenta praevia is associated with multiple pregnancy and previous lower segment scar. Manual removal of the placenta is not a risk for placenta praevia.

26. **(a)** False
    (b) False
    (c) False
    (d) True
    (e) True

27. **(a)** False
    (b) True
    (c) True
    (d) True
    (e) True

28. **(a)** False
    (b) False
    (c) False
    (d) True
    (e) False
    There is no proof that aspirin precipitates pulmonary embolism.

29. **(a)** False
    (b) True
    (c) True
    (d) False
    (e) False
    There is no association between the sex of the fetus and the incidence of this condition is approximately 1/1000 pregnancies.

30. **(a)** True
    (b) True
    (c) True
    (d) True
    (e) False

31. **(a)** True
    (b) True
    (c) False

(d) False
(e) True

32. (a) False
   (b) True
   (c) True
   (d) False
   (e) False

33. (a) True
   (b) True
   (c) True
   (d) True
   (e) False

34. (a) True
   (b) False
   (c) False
   (d) False
   (e) False
   Bed-rest has not been shown to be of any value in helping women with recurrent miscarriage. Aspirin and heparin are used in the treatment of immunological aetiology such as anti-cardiolipin syndrome but there is no conclusive evidence that it prevents the disease. Overall incidence is about 1%.

35. (a) True
   (b) False
   (c) False
   (d) True
   (e) True
   There is no evidence that urethral carbuncles are pre-cancerous.

36. (a) True
   (b) False
   (c) True
   (d) False
   (e) True
   Uterine fibroids may be symptomatic. GnRH analogues are currently used to shrink the size of these fibroids. Pressure by these fibroids may lead to back, renal or bowel problems.

37. (a) False
   (b) True
   (c) True

(d) True
(e) False
There is no relation to ethnic group.

38. **(a)** True
    (b) True
    (c) True
    (d) False
    (e) True

39. **(a)** False
    (b) False
    (c) False
    (d) True
    (e) True

40. **(a)** True
    (b) False
    (c) False
    (d) True
    (e) True
    High parity and an older age group, with an increase in intra-abdominal pressure, are known aetiological factors for genuine stress incontinence.

41. **(a)** True
    (b) False
    (c) False
    (d) False
    (e) True

42. **(a)** False
    (b) True
    (c) False
    (d) False
    (e) True
    Only 10% of cases of anti-D antibodies arise from failure to give prophylaxis. Women with a Rh negative blood group could always be followed up in the community but should any antibodies or titre increase they should be referred to hospital. Only 1% of Rh negative women become sensitized during pregnancy.

43. **(a)** True
    (b) False
    (c) True
    (d) True
    (e) .True

44. (a) True
    (b) True
    (c) True
    (d) True
    (e) True

45. (a) True
    (b) True
    (c) True
    (d) True
    (e) True

46. (a) False
    (b) True
    (c) True
    (d) True
    (e) False
The virus does influence the mode of delivery. Vertical transmission does occur but the incidence changes from one study to another. Although many units encourage screening for a 'high-risk' group the policy varies and in future it will be routine, although dependent on budgets and prevalence of the disease.

47. (a) True
    (b) True
    (c) False
    (d) True
    (e) False
There is a definite increase in congenital abnormalities in diabetics when they are pregnant as well as polyhydramnios and retinopathy. There is no evidence that jaundice is linked to diabetes in pregnancy.

48. (a) False
    (b) False
    (c) False
    (d) False
    (e) False
You must be up to date with the recent studies.

49. (a) True
    (b) True
    (c) False
    (d) True
    (e) True

50. (a) True
    (b) True
    (c) False
    (d) True
    (e) False
    Congenital dislocation of the hip is better diagnosed using ultrasound.
    There is no scientific evidence that it is related to the presence of other
    congenital abnormalities.

51. (a) True
    (b) False
    (c) True
    (d) True
    (e) False
    The condition is commoner in multiparous women. The diagnosis is
    usually made clinically, so there is no need to confirm it with ultrasound
    scan.

52. (a) False
    (b) True
    (c) True
    (d) True
    (e) False
    The prolapse of the umbilical cord complicates any malpresentation. It
    is commoner with breech.

53. (a) True
    (b) True
    (c) False
    (d) True
    (e) False
    Ulcerative colitis and inflammatory bowel disease lead to diarrhoea
    rather than vomiting.

54. (a) True
    (b) True
    (c) False
    (d) True
    (e) False
    The disease is commoner is social classes I and II.

55. (a) False
    (b) True
    (c) True
    (d) True
    (e) False

Infertility may be a sequela of severe endometriosis. There is no association with endometrial cancer in later life.

56. (a) False
(b) False
(c) True
(d) False
(e) False
Hysteroscopy can be easily done as an outpatient procedure under local anaesthesia. It is not contraindicated in a woman with a previous history of pelvic inflammatory disease.

57. (a) False
(b) True
(c) False
(d) False
(e) True
Retroversion occurs in about 20% of women. It leads to urinary retention from stretching of the urethra.

58. (a) True
(b) True
(c) True
(d) True
(e) True

59. (a) False
(b) False
(c) True
(d) False
(e) True
Ovarian cysts in pregnancy vary in origin. Corpus luteal cysts account for 70% where dermoid accounts for only 5%. Very rarely malignant ovarian cysts occur in pregnancy. Torsion of the cyst occurs in pregnancy and sometimes bleeding into the cyst. Obstruction is a rare occurrence of an ovarian cyst in pregnancy.

60. (a) True
(b) True
(c) True
(d) True
(e) True

61. (a) True
(b) True

(c) True
(d) False
(e) True
Applying selective criteria and with the agreement of the parents, breech presentation may be delivered vaginally.

62. (a) True
    (b) True
    (c) True
    (d) True
    (e) True

63. (a) True
    (b) True
    (c) True
    (d) True
    (e) True

64. (a) True
    (b) False
    (c) True
    (d) False
    (e) True
Maternal pyrexia and tachycardia as well as fetal tachycardia are all indicative of chorioamnionitis.

65. (a) True
    (b) False
    (c) False
    (d) True
    (e) True
In cleft palate feeding problems can develop and, therefore, special teats are needed. Surgery to correct cleft palate is best done at around 1 year.

66. (a) False
    (b) False
    (c) False
    (d) True
    (e) True
The incidence of a diaphragmatic hernia is 1/4000; 90% of cases occur on the left side through the posterolateral foramen of Bochdalek.

67. (a) True
    (b) True
    (c) True

(d) True

(e) True

68. (a) True

(b) True

(c) True

(d) True

(e) True

NOTES ON GYNAECOLOGY

4

HISTORY AND EXAMINATION IN GYNAECOLOGY

Taking the history

It is essential to gain the patient's trust and to allow her to express her concerns and feelings.

Following the initial introduction between yourself and the patient it is often useful to ask a standard set of questions such as her age, date of birth, the first day of her last menstrual period, the type of contraception she is using and the date of her last cervical smear. Following this you should put your pen down, sit back and ask the patient to describe her symptoms.

The presenting symptom or chief complaint is one of the most important aspects of *any* gynaecological history.

The gynaecological history must be detailed and obtained in a sensitive, sympathetic and objective manner. It is essential to keep a record of the main symptom(s) and the duration of each symptom. If the patient has pain then you should elucidate the following characteristics concerning the nature of the pain:

- Site
- Radiation
- Character
- Severity
- Duration
- Periodicity
- Aggravating factors
- Relieving factors
- Temporal change

If the patient is complaining of menstrual irregularity it is essential to determine what her usual menstrual cycle was and how and when it changed. The menstrual cycle is most often expressed as two numbers X/Y where the numerator (X) refers to the number of days of bleeding and the denominator (Y) refers to the number of days between the onset of menstruation in successive cycles. If the rhythm is variable it is conventional to express Y as a range such as 14–28, or 56–72.

If the patient complains of infertility you must establish the frequency of coitus, whether or not there are any specific problems associated with coitus and the attitude of each partner to pregnancy.

Standard questions include the age at menarche, contraceptive history, history of cervical smears, history of pelvic sepsis (if any) and whether or not the patient has previously undergone gynaecological surgery.

A relevant *family history* must be taken.

The patient's *obstetric history* is essential. You need to establish the number of pregnancies she has had, the number of living children she has and you must be able to explain any difference between the number of pregnancies and the number of living children. For example a patient may have experienced previous miscarriages, termination of pregnancy, ectopic pregnancy, stillbirth or the loss of a live-born child.

If a patient has suffered a previous miscarriage or termination of pregnancy you need to ascertain exactly what happened and why.

If a patient has previously undergone gynaecological surgery – such as a suction termination of pregnancy – you must enquire as to where the operation was performed and whether or not there were any complications.

The importance of the *medical history* simply cannot be over-emphasized. In addition to details of serious illnesses, debilitating conditions and surgical history you must enquire about a history of blood transfusion, the current list of medications the patient is using and a history of drug sensitivity.

Personal history: enquire about your patient's partner – age, current relationship and state of health; the patient's occupation; the effect of her present condition on her occupation. The level of consumption of cigarettes and alcohol (if any) must be documented.

At the end of the history it is often useful to write down a brief summary of exactly why the patient has come to see you, what her own perception of her condition is and her expectations for treatment. For example a patient who suffers from secondary amenorrhoea due to hyperprolactinaemia may not necessarily be concerned about anovulatory infertility. The patient may simply be concerned about what has happened to her menstrual blood loss. Another patient with an excessive vaginal discharge and a perfectly normal cervical smear may have a close friend who is undergoing surgical treatment for a pre-malignant condition of the cervix. Under such circumstances the patient may be consulting you in order to seek reassurance that all is well.

The following key symptoms and signs should alert you to certain conditions until proven otherwise.

- Post-menopausal bleeding—malignancy in the pelvis
- Post-coital bleeding—lesion in the cervix
- Abdominal distension in a middle-aged or elderly woman—ovarian tumour
- Ulcer in the labia of an elderly woman—vulval cancer

Gynaecological examination

Examine the patient as a whole person and measure her height, weight, pulse rate and blood pressure.

- You must be able to assess the pallor of the mucus membranes, the presence or absence of jaundice, whether or not the patient is breathless and whether or not there are variations in the colour of her skin and tongue that would indicate the presence of conditions such as cyanosis.
- Examine the abdomen with the patient lying flat and the abdomen exposed from the suprapubic area to the xiphisternum with the patient's arms by her side.
- *Inspect the abdomen*: this point *cannot* be over-emphasized. You must check for any obvious distension, the presence of surgical scars, abnormal pigmentation of the skin and male-type distribution of hair.
- Palpate the abdomen, including groin, loins and hernial orifices.
- Perform a pelvic examination with the patient remaining adequately covered in the presence of a female chaperone (for instance a nurse) and using an adequate source of light.
- Inspect the introitus and perineum and check for the following: erythema, labial symmetry, appearance of the clitoris, position of the urethra, atrophy, genital warts, genital ulceration, any swelling in the Bartholin's glands or paraurethral glands, obvious signs of genitourinary prolapse, perineal scarring and leucoplakia.
- Pass an appropriate speculum. Cusco's bivalve speculum is passed with the patient in the dorsal position while a Sim's speculum may be passed with the patient lying in the left lateral position.
- Inspect the vagina and cervix and take a cervical smear if required. With the patient's consent you may take an endocervical swab for the detection of *Chlamydia trachomatis* and *Neisseria gonorrhoeae* and a high vaginal swab for trichomons vaginalis, evidence of bacterial vaginosis, candida culture, measurement of vaginal pH and microscopy.
- Withdraw the speculum gently.
- Perform a bimanual examination of the pelvis with the patient in the dorsal position. You must check for tenderness on moving the cervix, the position of the cervix, the nature of the cervical os, and whether it is small or patulous.
- Assess the size of the uterus, and whether or not it is anteverted, axial or retroverted.
- Palpate the adnexa for tenderness and masses.
- A rectal examination should be considered if your patient either has or is suspected of suffering from a malignant lesion.
- A rectal examination is often useful in assessing a patient with a rectocele.

At the end of the examination it is important to offer the patient some clean tissues and to allow adequate time and privacy for her to get dressed again.

PHYSIOLOGY OF MENSTRUATION

Menstruation occurs as a result of the response of the endometrium to hormonal changes in a woman's body. The menstrual flow itself consists of blood, mucus and endometrial cells. There are wide natural variations in the duration of menstruation and in the length of the menstrual cycle. It is standard practice to express the menstrual cycle as two numbers, X/Y. X refers to the duration of the menstrual bleeding and Y refers to the period of time in days between the first day of menstruation and the last day in the cycle before bleeding occurs in the subsequent cycle. Although it is commonly held that women with a 4/28 cycle have a 'normal' cycle, in practice the cycle is very variable. The following points are useful from a clinical point of view:

- A change in a woman's menstrual cycle is often significant.
- X is usually influenced by local factors within the female genital tract such as the presence of a sub-mucous fibroid, endometrial polyp or an intrauterine contraceptive device.
- Y is often influenced by systemic and hormonal factors.
- The average menstrual blood loss is approximately 80 ml, although it must be borne in mind that a visual estimation of blood loss is notoriously difficult.
- The presence of fibrinolytic systems in the endometrium prevents the formation of blood clots. If the patient passes blood clots it is clear that the bleeding for that particular woman is exceeding the capacity of the fibrinolytic systems in the endometrium.

Hormonal changes

Fig. 4.1 shows the changes in the levels of serum follicle stimulation hormone (FSH), luteinizing hormone (LH), oestrogen and progesterone over a hypothetical 28-day cycle. Day 1 indicates the onset of menstruation and in a woman with a 28-day cycle ovulation usually occurs on day 14. It is important to note, however, that a woman may have anovulatory cycles.

The 14 days prior to ovulation comprise the follicular phase and the period of time of 14 days following ovulation is called the luteal phase. The terms follicular and luteal refer to the ovarian follicles (see next section). The following changes occur in the hormones:

Serum FSH   This rises during the follicular phase of the menstrual cycle. The production of FSH from the anterior lobe of the pituitary gland is stimulated by gonadotrophin-releasing hormones (GnRH) from the hypothalamus. Follicle stimulation hormone stimulates the growth and maturation of the Graafian follicles in the ovary. The secretion of FSH from the anterior lobe of the pituitary is inhibited by a rise in serum oestrogen

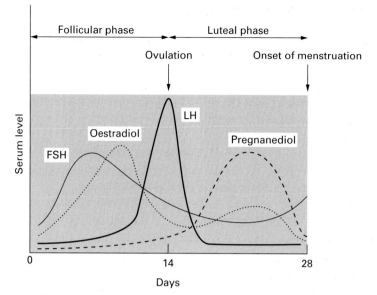

Fig. 4.1 This schematic diagram indicates the changes in serum FSH, LH, oestradiol and pregnanediol levels in a woman with a 28-day cycle who is in the reproductive age group. During the follicular phase the serum oestradiol rises in response to rising serum FSH and then the negative feedback of oestradiol on the hypothalamic–pituitary axis leads to a fall in the serum FSH. The pre-ovulatory surge in serum LH is necessary for ovulation to occur. The rise in serum pregnanediol and the (smaller) rise in estradiol during the luteal phase represent production of those two hormones in the corpus luteum of the ovary. The corpus luteum regresses after 10–14 days and hence the serum oestradiol and pregnanediol levels fall and menstruation occurs.

and this is one of the classic examples of negative feedback in human medicine.

Serum LH   Luteinizing hormone is produced in the anterior lobe of the pituitary gland and its production and secretion are stimulated by GnRH. There is a pre-ovulatory surge of serum LH which occurs in response to a rise in serum oestrogen levels. The sharp rise in serum LH initiates ovulation.

Serum oestrogen   Oestrogen is produced in the ovarian Graafian follicles in response to follicle stimulation hormone. During the follicular phase of the cycle the serum oestrogen rises steadily as shown in Fig. 4.1. However the serum oestrogen falls prior to ovulation. The rise in serum oestrogen during the luteal phase of the cycle is due to production of oestrogen by the corpus luteum.

Progesterone   The serum progesterone is low during the follicular phase of the cycle but rises significantly during the luteal phase of the cycle. Progesterone is produced in the corpus luteum and the fall in serum progesterone prior to menstruation reflects the degeneration of the corpus luteum.

The ovary

The Graafian follicles in the ovary enlarge and mature in response to FSH. However many ovarian follicles undergo a process of atresia and one follicle (occasionally more than one) enlarges over the course of the follicular phase, ruptures and releases the ovum on day 14 in a 28-day cycle. It is important to note that the follicular phase of the cycle is far more variable than the luteal phase. The latter lasts approximately 14 days. Following ovulation the Graafian follicle becomes a corpus luteum. Over the 14 days of the luteal phase of the cycle the corpus luteum secretes oestrogen and progesterone and then degenerates and is reabsorbed within the ovary. Occasionally a cyst of the corpus luteum may develop.

The endometrium

Following menstruation the endometrium has a 'resting phase' lasting for a day or so. Regenerative changes occur in both the endometrial glands and stroma within 3–4 days of the onset of menstruation. During the follicular phase of the cycle the endometrium proliferates and mitoses are observed in both the glandular epithelium and the stroma. As a result of endometrial proliferation the endometrial glands appear to be narrow (on light microscopic examination) and they are lined by multi-layered non-secretory epithelium; this is the reason why the follicular phase is sometimes termed the proliferative phase of the cycle. Following ovulation the endometrium is said to be in the secretory phase and both glandular secretion and stromal differentiation are observed. Over a period of approximately 4 days the endometrial glands increase in diameter and become tortuous. Sub-nuclear glycogen containing vacuoles may be observed in the glandular epithelium and it is generally held that the presence of sub-nuclear vacuoles in all of the cells of at least 50% of the endometrial glands is histological evidence of ovulation. From the 5th day after ovulation glandular secretion by the endometrium reaches a peak and the glands become tortuous. Subsequently the endometrium becomes even more tortuous and glandular secretion decreases. The spiral arterioles of the endometrium are well developed at this stage. Towards the end of the secretory phase the endometrial stroma is infiltrated by granulated lymphocytes and polymorphonuclear neutrophils. Menstruation is characterized by endometrial crumbling, necrosis and haemorrhage. It is important to note that the basal layer of the endometrium is not shed at menstruation and remains to enter a fresh proliferative phase during the next cycle.

The cervix

From the clinical perspective the most significant change in the cervix is seen in the cervical mucus around about the time of ovulation. There is an increase in cervical secretion and the cervical mucus becomes more fluid. Within a day or so of ovulation the cervical mucus becomes more viscous.

The Fallopian tubes

The epithelial lining of the Fallopian tubes undergoes cyclical change. During the follicular phase the epithelium increases in height. At the time of ovulation the ciliated cells lining the lumen of the Fallopian tubes are well developed and the cilia beat in waves in the direction of the uterus. During the luteal phase the secretory cells lining the lumen of the Fallopian tubes become more developed while the ciliated cells regress.

The vagina

The vaginal epithelium thickens during the follicular phase of the cycle and the individual cells mature just prior to ovulation. During the luteal phase inhibition of squamous maturation occurs and marked exfoliation of cells may be observed.

PUBERTY

The age at which a young woman has her first menstrual period is termed the menarche and the period of time around the menarche is termed puberty. Puberty is characterized by certain morphological changes in the female body and these are the changes in secondary sexual characteristics.

Changes at puberty

The following signs appear:

- Growth in height
- Development and growth of the breasts
- Development and growth of pubic hair
- Development and growth of axillary hair
- First menstrual period

Growth and development of the breasts are usually seen between the ages of 8 and 13 years with an average of approximately 11 years. The age at menarche has been falling in recent years, certainly in industrialized countries. Most females in the United Kingdom would reach the menarche between the ages of 10 and 15 years and the average age is probably 12. It is important for the GP to note that menstruation may sometimes occur prior to the growth and development of axillary or even pubic hair. The first few cycles following the menarche are usually anovulatory.

Precocious sexual development

Precocious sexual development is defined as menstruation prior to the age of 10 or development and growth of the breasts and pubic hair prior to the age of 8 years. The causes of precocious sexual development in a female are as follows:

1. Constitutional
2. Intracranial lesion, cerebral tumour, encephalitis, meningitis
3. Albright's syndrome constituting precocious puberty, polyostotic fibrous dysplasia and café-au-lait spots on the skin
4. Oestrogen-secreting tumour of the ovary.

Any female with precocious sexual development should be referred to a specialist or (preferably) a paediatric gynaecologist for investigation and management.

Delayed puberty

A female develops secondary sexual characteristics in response to endogenous oestrogen. If a young woman has normal secondary sexual characteristics you may safely conclude that the body's oestrogen environment is normal, therefore a young woman with normal secondary sexual characteristics who presents with concern that she has not yet commenced menstruation may be reassured up until the age of 16 years. The most common cause of delayed puberty is constitutional. However, a young woman who has absent secondary sexual characteristics warrants further investigations at the age of 14 years.

Dysmenorrhoea

Early menstrual cycles may be irregular, heavy and painful. As a generalization ovulatory cycles lead to dysmenorrhoea, whereas anovulatory cycles are associated with pain-free menstruation. If a young woman attends your surgery with symptoms of dysmenorrhoea, menorrhagia and irregular menstruation at puberty it is important to listen carefully and sympathetically. Management should include an explanation of the physiology of menstruation and the prescription of simple, non-habit forming analgesics. In more severe cases the combined oral contraceptive pill may be used to control the menstrual cycle.

Vaginal bleeding in childhood

The causes of this distressing symptom include the following:

1. Precocious sexual development
2. Foreign body in the vagina
3. Tumours of the genital tract
4. Non-accidental injury
5. Trauma to the genital tract.

An examination under anaesthesia may sometimes be necessary in order to identify and remove a foreign body. Fortunately tumours of the genital tract during childhood are very rare. Sarcoma botryoides is a rare tumour which occurs during childhood and arises from the sub-epithelial tissues of the vagina or cervix. The lesion is grape-like in appearance and treatment with radical surgery and chemotherapy is necessary. It is important to remember that grape-like vaginal polyps in childhood are more likely to be caused by sarcoma botryoides (itself very rare) rather than simple benign polypi.

AMENORRHOEA

Amenorrhoea is defined as absent menstruation for longer than 6 consecutive months. Amenorrhoea may be temporary or permanent, physiological or pathological. Primary amenorrhoea is amenorrhoea that occurs in a young woman who has not as yet had her first menstrual period. It is standard practice to consider further investigations in a young woman who has primary amenorrhoea in the presence of normal secondary sexual characteristics at the age of 16 years or who has primary amenorrhoea in the absence of normal secondary sexual characteristics by the age of 14 years (see p. 92).

Physiological causes of secondary amenorrhoea include pregnancy, lactation and the menopause.

Significance
The prevalence of amenorrhoea in the female population is approximately 2% (excluding physiological causes of secondary amenorrhoea). The general practitioner is therefore well advised to have a firm grasp of the basic principles of the management of women with amenorrhoea; furthermore, it is important to note that some causes of amenorrhoea may be potentially fatal.

Causes
For normal menstruation to occur the hypothalamic–pituitary–ovarian axis should be normal, the uterus – and in particular the endometrium – must be healthy and the cervix and vagina must be patent (see p. 88). The function of the higher centres in the central nervous system, the cerebral cortex, the adrenal gland and the woman's chromosomes all play a part in influencing menstruation. The causes of primary amenorrhoea are shown in Box 4.1.

Turner's syndrome (45 XO) is the most common cause of gonadal dysgenesis. The affected patient has short stature, webbing of the neck, widely-spaced nipples, cardiac malformations (aortic coarctation is usual but there may be other malformations) and renal abnormalities. Premature ovarian failure is the rule in women with Turner's syndrome although spontaneous menstruation and (very rarely) fertility have been reported.

In haemotocolpos the patient has an intact hymen which actually covers the introitus without affecting micturition. The vagina distends with

Box 4.1   Causes of primary amenorrhoea

- Primary ovarian failure: gonadal dysgenesis
- Congenital abnormalities: haematocolpos, Müllerian agenesis
- Intersex: true testicular feminization syndrome due to androgen receptor insensitivity, 5-alpha reductase deficiency leading to male pseudohermaphroditism
- Late-onset congenital adrenal hyperplasia
- Hypogonadotrophic hypogonadism
- Hypopituitarism
- Polycystic ovarian syndrome
- Other causes: weight-related amenorrhoea and hyperprolactinaemia

It should go without saying that pregnancy must be considered in all women who have amenorrhoea

menstrual blood and the patient often complains of severe dysmenorrhoea. In patients with Müllerian agenesis the vagina ends in a blind loop, the cervix and uterus are missing but the ovaries appear to be normal.

The endocrinological causes of primary amenorrhoea are listed in Box 4.2 but it is important to note that hypogonadotrophic hypogonadism may occur secondary to tumours within the central nervous system such as craniopharyngioma, germinoma, glioma and dermoid cysts. Isolated deficiency of GnRH secretion associated with the absence of smell and colour-blindness constitute Kallman's syndrome, which is an autosomal dominant condition. It is important for the GP to note that the conditions which may lead to primary amenorrhoea may also be classified according to whether or not secondary sexual development is present or deficient. Gonadal dysgenesis, 5-alpha reductase deficiency, congenital adrenal hyperplasia (late onset) and hypogonadatrophic hypogonadism are associated with poorly developed secondary sexual characteristics. By contrast haematocolpos, Müllerian agenesis, true testicular feminization syndrome secondary to androgen receptor insensitivity and polycystic ovarian syndrome would be associated with the normal development of secondary sexual characteristics.

It is important to recognize that (a) the causes of amenorrhoea are very varied; and (b) some of them such as anorexia nervosa and major systemic illnesses are potentially fatal.

Management

The diagnosis and treatment of primary and secondary amenorrhoea are best left to a specialist. Indeed for several of the conditions which have been listed the services of a tertiary referral centre with a team of paediatric gynaecologists, urological surgeons, psychosexual counsellors, endocrinologists, pathologists and appropriately trained nurses would be

Box 4.2   Causes of secondary amenorrhoea (pathological)

- Endocrinological causes: hyperprolactinaemia, polycystic ovarian syndrome, premature ovarian failure, hypogonadotrophic hypogonadism, hypopituitarism
- Weight-related amenorrhoea
- Anorexia nervosa
- Exercise-induced amenorrhoea
- Psychological stress
- Asherman's syndrome
- Cervical stenosis
- Systemic disease, malignancy, virilizing tumours of the adrenal gland, tuberculosis, involuntary starvation

mandatory. However the GP plays a pivotal role in the initial screening and diagnosis of patients. The following checklist will help you to arrive at a reasonable working diagnosis and decision on where to refer the patient.

1. A full history, including social history, is important and you must be in a position to answer the following questions: does the patient suffer from stress? Has she undergone gynaecological surgery which may have produced cervical stenosis? Has the patient been exposed to or is she currently taking any hormone therapy? What is the patient's attitude to her fertility?
2. What is the patient's weight and height? As a generalization, Turner's syndrome or pan-hypopituitarism may be suspected in a 16-year-old who is 1.47 metres tall or less.
3. On physical examination are there any features of virilization? Are the secondary sexual characteristics well developed? Is the lower genital tract normal?
4. Basic investigations: karyotype, endocrine profile, ultrasound examination of the pelvis.

The long-term management of women with amenorrhoea depends both on the underlying cause and on the long-term effects of oestrogen deficiency.

In many women amenorrhoea may resolve spontaneously. In the case of women with Turner's syndrome referral to an appropriate sub-specialist centre is essential, so that patients may receive counselling concerning options for fertility that include the possibility of oocyte donation and assisted conception. Hormone replacement therapy would also need to be considered. Patients suffering from haematocolpos would need to undergo a simple operation where a cruciate incision is performed on the hymen under general anaesthesia. The operation is simple to perform and the results are excellent but the patient will need adequate counselling. Patients with polycystic ovarian syndrome should be managed accordingly (see below) and patients with anorexia nervosa need the help of a consultant psychiatrist.

The long-term effects of oestrogen deficiency in women with untreated primary or secondary amenorrhoea include the following:

- Increased risk of osteoporosis
- Increased risk of cardiovascular disease
- Infertility
- Impaired sexuality

Long-term hormone replacement therapy would need to be considered for many women once the underlying cause for the amenorrhoea has been established. Prolonged oestrogen deficiency leads to atrophic changes in the lower genital tract which will contribute to superficial dyspareunia and decreased libido. The issue of fertility requires detailed counselling and discussion. Recent advances in technology have led to the options of oocyte donation, surrogacy and reconstructive pelvic surgery.

The presence of a Y chromosome in a patient with gonadal dysgenesis increases the risk of malignant change in the gonad. Under such circumstances bilateral gonadectomy would need to be considered.

POLYCYSTIC OVARIAN SYNDROME

Polycystic ovarian syndrome (PCOS) is the most common cause of oligomenorrhoea (infrequent periods), anovulatory infertility and hirsutism. The condition is one of the most common problems encountered in reproductive endocrinology, and the general practitioner must understand the prevalence of the condition, its basic pathophysiology, its impact on women's lives and the principles for treatment.

Pathophysiology
There are three main endocrinological abnormalities and hence the condition has sometimes been referred to as the 'vicious tricycle'. The endocrine abnormalities are as follows:

1. Elevated pituitary derived serum luteinizing hormone (LH)
2. An increase in the ovarian secretion of serum androstenedione and serum testosterone
3. Dysfunction of insulin receptors leading to hyperinsulinaemia.

Increased secretion of LH leads to increased activity of the ovarian stromal tissues and disordered hormone production within the ovary. This leads to acyclical production of oestrogens from the ovary and the production of LH by the anterior lobe of the pituitary gland is stimulated further. The serum FSH is usually normal in patients with PCOS. The ovaries are usually enlarged and have a characteristic ultrasound picture (see next section).

Using ultrasound criteria for diagnosis PCOS has been detected in over 50% of women with anovulation, over 90% of women with idiopathic hirsutism and approximately one-fifth of normal female volunteers. PCOS is therefore common.

Diagnosis

You should consider the diagnosis of PCOS in any woman who has anovulatory infertility, hirsutism, long cycles, obesity or diabetes mellitus. The diagnosis of PCOS rests on the combination of the clinical history, findings on examination, ultrasound criteria and the results of hormone assays.

The ultrasound criteria for the diagnosis of PCOS are as follows:

- Increased ovarian volume of more than 9 cm^3
- More than 10 follicles in each ovary with a diameter of 3–8 mm
- Increased stromal density

At least two of the three criteria must be fulfilled, and both transabdominal and transvaginal ultrasound examination may be necessary.

The endocrinological features of PCOS are as follows:

- Elevated serum LH
- Normal pre-menopausal serum FSH
- Elevated serum androstenedione
- Elevated serum testosterone
- Decreased serum sex-hormone binding globulin

It is important to note that not all patients with PCOS would exhibit all of the characteristic features. The decrease in the serum sex-hormone binding globulin will lead to an elevation in the free androgen index; the free androgens lead to the development of hirsutism against a background of genetic predisposition. For example Chinese women with PCOS are rarely hirsute whereas women from the Indian sub-continent would develop hirsutism more readily in the presence of PCOS.

Complications

It is important to note that PCOS has an impact on the overall health of the woman. Women with PCOS require careful counselling as they are at increased risk of the following:

- Diabetes mellitus
- Cardiovascular disease
- Hypertension
- Osteoporosis
- Endometrial neoplasia
- Recurrent abortion

Further research is essential in order to precisely determine the underlying pathophysiology and clinical interrelationships of PCOS and the conditions associated with it.

Treatment

The general practitioner has a crucial role to play in the diagnosis and counselling of women with PCOS. Its treatment is influenced by various factors including whether or not the patient wishes to conceive and has a history of infertility, her body weight, whether or not she is concerned about any hirsutism which may be present and the presence of complications. The treatment of PCOS is best left to a specialist.

Women who are overweight should be given advice on a weight-reducing diet. Anovulatory infertility is treated with clomifene. There have been some reports of success in the treatment of PCOS with laparoscopic ovarian 'drilling' using electrocautery.

HIRSUTISM

Definition

Hirsutism is defined as the excessive growth of human terminal hair; it is *not* the same as virilism. Virilism is rare, associated with an excessive amount of androgens in the female body, and its clinical signs include deepening of the voice, laryngomegaly, clitoral hypertrophy and hirsutism.

Hirsutism is commonly associated with menstrual disturbance, acne, seborrhoea and a male pattern of hair growth on the face, chest, lower abdomen and thighs.

Prevalence

The exact prevalence of hirsutism is unquantifiable as it is a subjective diagnosis. There are ethnic variations in the amount of growth of terminal hair and different women have different thresholds for what they find acceptable. If a woman complains to her GP that she has an excessive growth of hair then the problem must be investigated.

Pathophysiology

The growth of terminal hair is stimulated by androgens. In women androgen arises from three sources and they are as follows:

1. Peripheral conversion of androstenedione in the fat, liver and skin – 50%
2. The ovaries stimulated by serum LH – 25%
3. The adrenal glands stimulated by serum adrenocorticotrophin (ACTH) – 25%

Most of the testosterone which is produced in the female body is bound to serum sex-hormone binding globulin (SHBG). Free serum testosterone is converted by the enzyme 5-alpha reductase in the skin into dihydrotestosterone.

Dihydrotestosterone is a potent androgen which acts on the androgen receptors in the hair follicles. Various conditions including some medical drugs produce hyperandrogenaemia.

Causes

The following causes must be considered in any woman with hirsutism:

- Iatrogenic – the use of androgens, danazol, anabolic steroids, high doses of norethisterone
- Idiopathic
- Ovarian – polycystic ovarian syndrome, ovarian tumours such as testosterone secreting arrhenoblastoma and hyperthecosis of the ovary.
- Adrenal – congenital adrenal hyperplasia, Cushing's syndrome, virilizing tumours of the adrenal cortex such as adrenal carcinoma.

Diagnosis

The management of any clinical problem depends on the clinical methods of history taking, examination and basic investigations. Specific features in history taking for a woman with hirsutism should include the history of exactly how long the patient has noticed increased hair growth and how quickly it is developing. It is also important to elucidate the patient's menstrual history, history of drug ingestion and whether or not there is a history of infertility. On examination you must note the extent of hair growth, the presence of acne, features of virilism and the patient's body weight.

Specific investigations should be aimed at diagnosing or excluding PCOS (see p. 96). Congenital adrenal hyperplasia of late onset is a very rare cause of hirsutism and should be considered following failure of standard treatment (see below). Most cases of congenital adrenal hyperplasia present with ambiguous genitalia at birth and are usually diagnosed during childhood. A patient with Cushing's syndrome would have hirsutism, Cushingoid striae, hypertension and 'central' obesity. A virilized patient with an elevated serum testosterone may have a virilizing tumour such as adrenal carcinoma. 'Idiopathic' hirsutism is a diagnosis by exclusion.

The general practitioner should be familiar with patients' reactions to excessive hair growth, the pathophysiology of hirsutism and the importance of establishing an individual patient's androgen status. Further management of the hirsute patient and especially the virilized patient is best left to a specialist.

Treatment

The treatment of hirsutism depends on the underlying cause. 'Idiopathic' hirsutism and women with PCOS may be offered the following options:

- A weight-reducing diet. Approximately one-half of the androgens in a woman's body arise from peripheral conversion of oestrogens to androgens; if a woman loses weight then the level of endogenous androgen production decreases.
- Cosmetic options include shaving, bleaching, plucking and electrolysis.
- Medical treatment. A combination of oestrogen, ethinylestradiol with the anti-androgen and progestogen cyproterone acetate is a highly effective regimen. Ethinylestradiol decreases the effect of serum LH on the ovary and stimulates production of SHBG in the liver. These mechanisms lead to a decrease in the level of free serum testosterone. Cyproterone acetate acts as an androgen receptor blocker at the level of the dihydrotestosterone receptor in hair follicles. It is important to note that the combination of ethinylestradiol and cyproterone acetate leads to a decrease in hirsutism over a period of approximately 6–18 months. The patient should *not* be pregnant when she starts taking the treatment and the treatment is in itself an effective contraceptive. Side effects include deranged liver function. Paradoxically the patient may develop acne although this rapidly resolves.

PRE-MENSTRUAL TENSION

Pre-menstrual tension is a well-defined disease of variable severity affecting women in their reproductive years. It is widely prevalent.

Diagnosis

Pre-menstrual tension (PMT) is characterized by physical, emotional and behavioural symptoms which tend to appear 7–10 days prior to menstruation. The symptoms tend to disappear within the first day or two of the start of menses. Box 4.3 lists symptoms which may appear with PMT. The diagnosis of PMT depends on a careful and sympathetic case history followed by a physical examination in order to establish that the patient's

---

Box 4.3   Symptoms of pre-menstrual tension

Physical	Lower abdominal pain
	Lower abdominal distension
	Fluid retention with peripheral oedema
	Mild weight gain
Emotional	Irritability
	Lassitude
	Depressed affect
Behavioural	Craving for certain types of food such as chocolate
	Obsessive tendencies

---

pelvis is normal. It is thought that the symptoms of PMT are produced during the luteal phase of the menstrual cycle by cyclical ovarian activity.

Counselling

One of the most important issues in the management of patients with PMT is the acknowledgement by the doctor that the patient is suffering from a discrete disorder. Women have often read about 'PMT' or 'pre-menstrual syndrome' in popular magazines and newspapers. It is vital that you acknowledge the patient's symptoms and her concern and provide her with an explanation of the disorder and how it is diagnosed.

Treatment

All women require explanation and reassurance. For some this may well be all that is required. However some women may actually require surgical intervention depending on the severity of the symptoms, age, attitude to fertility and any co-existing illnesses. Options for treatment are listed in Box 4.4.

If these options fail it is essential to refer the patient to a specialist for further advice and help. The options available to the specialist include:

1. The use of gonadorelin-releasing hormone therapy in the form of intramuscular injections of goserelin or leuprorelin every 4 weeks together with 'add back' hormone replacement therapy.
2. Total abdominal hysterectomy and bilateral salpingo-oophorectomy followed by oestrogen replacement therapy.

It is important to note that the use of GnRH analogues is associated with the development of menopausal symptoms and osteoporosis. That is the reason why 'add back' hormone replacement therapy is also offered at the same time. Neither of these preparations provide contraception and so it is

---

Box 4.4   Options for treatment of PMT

- Counselling and reassurance
- Advice on the use of evening primrose oil which may affect metabolism of fatty acids
- Vitamin B6 (pyridoxine) tablets may be purchased over the counter. However concern has been expressed over the risk of neuropathy with prolonged therapy
- Progesterone (for example in the form of vaginal pessary) given during the luteal phase of the cycle
- A low-dose oestrogen (for example transdermal estradiol used in hormone replacement therapy) during the follicular phase of the cycle
- The combined oral contraceptive pill
- Danazol – note side effects may be very unpleasant

---

important to counsel the woman that a reliable method of contraception must also be used. The concurrent use of 'add back' hormone replacement therapy would obviate many of the unpleasant menopausal side effects of the GnRH analogue and prevent the development of osteoporosis. Data are available to support the use of this form of treatment over a 6-month period but there are few data (at the present time) to support this particular measure as an option for the long term.

A few patients may well require total abdominal hysterectomy and bilateral salpingo-oophorectomy followed by hormone replacement therapy. Such patients require detailed counselling by a specialist. It is important to emphasize to the woman that the symptoms of a premature menopause following bilateral oophorectomy may be as crippling as the symptoms of severe PMT. The operation of total abdominal hysterectomy and bilateral salpingo-oophorectomy in a young women is an extremely serious undertaking. The relief of menopausal symptoms by giving oestrogen replacement therapy to a young woman who has undergone bilateral oophorectomy may be difficult to achieve. Consultation with a specialist is essential if the woman has severe PMT and surgery is being considered.

INFECTIONS OF THE FEMALE GENITAL TRACT

Infections of the female genital tract are a common cause of the problems that bring a woman to her GP. Although a small amount of vaginal discharge is perfectly normal in many women the symptom of a malodorous vaginal discharge may occur in the three most prevalent infections of the lower genital tract: candidiasis (monilia), vaginal trichomoniasis and bacterial vaginosis. There are several other causes of infection in the female genital tract and these include chlamydial infection of the cervix, gonococcal infection and genital wart virus infection. It is important to realize that infection of the lower genital tract may well be associated with infection in the upper genital tract and extra-genital sites. For example syphilis, which is a bacterial infection caused by the organism *Treponema pallidum*, causes florid manifestations which may well influence the genital tract as well as systemic infection which may not be recognized for several years.

One of the most important distinctions to make in the clinical microbiology of the female genital tract is to differentiate between a sexually *transmitted* disease and a sexually *transmissible* disease. A sexually transmitted disease is caused by an organism which can only be sexually transmitted and examples include *Chlamydia trachomatis* and *Neisseria gonorrhoeae*. Organisms which are sexually transmissible but may also give rise to opportunistic infections include monilia and anaerobic or bacterial vaginosis. It is important to realize that some conditions require referral to a specialist in genitourinary medicine. A patient who has a sexually transmitted disease must be referred to a genitourinary clinic; the advantages of such a referral are as follows:

- Management by a specialist
- Expert counselling is available
- A full range of swabs and facilities for investigations
- Contact tracing for certain conditions may be carried out.

The woman herself may feel that there is a degree of stigma associated with attending a genitourinary medicine clinic. Furthermore, she may be familiar with the GP's surgery and prefer not have to travel in order to receive further advice, investigations and treatment. It is important to raise these points in discussion and to acknowledge the patient's own feelings and concerns; however, it is essential to refer patients with sexually transmitted diseases to a clinic.

Role of the laboratory

A microbiology laboratory can provide all the swabs, materials and transport media necessary for you to take the appropriate swabs. It is extremely important that each specimen is labelled correctly with an appropriate request form for investigation. Transport of specimens to the laboratory must be prompt and reliable. The laboratory should ensure that the appropriate investigation is carried out for the appropriate organism. Please remember that the results of investigations for infectious diseases of the female genital tract have medical as well as social implications: for example, a patient who has chlamydial infection of the cervix may well ask you how she acquired the infection; the doctor who is managing the patient (GP, gynaecologist or specialist in genitourinary medicine) must be certain of the diagnosis from a scientific point of view. It would be incorrect to make a clinical diagnosis of, say, chlamydial or gonococcal infection of the cervix. In the example of infection with *Chlamydia trachomatis* the laboratory would process the appropriate specimen using either an immunofluorescent microscopic technique or enzyme-linked immunosorbant assay (ELISA). If a specimen is identified as 'positive' then further material from the same swab would be analysed for *Chlamydia trachomatis* using either a polymerase chain reaction (PCR) or cell culture in order to confirm the diagnosis beyond any reasonable doubt.

History and examination

A full history must be taken with special reference to the duration of the symptoms, the nature of the vaginal discharge (if any), whether or not there is any odour associated with the discharge, previous history of genital tract infection, the health of the woman's partner, her occupation, social habits, current medications and history of allergy to drugs. The presence of associated medical conditions must be noted down. *The possibility of pregnancy must also be considered.*

On clinical examination you must look for the following:

- Genital ulcers
- Genital warts
- Swellings of the Bartholin's gland with evidence of inflammation
- Condylomata
- Pubic lice
- Vaginitis
- The appearance of the cervix
- Pelvic tenderness on bimanual palpation
- Cervical excitation
- 'Hotness' of the vagina

The term vaginitis implies redness of the vaginal mucosa and swelling of the mucus membrane; petechiae may also be present. The cervix may contain a simple ectopy or a hypertrophic ectopy. The cervical mucus may be clear, cloudy or mucopurulent. The presence of mucopurulent cervical mucus has been considered as the equivalent of a purulent urethritis in men. However it would be unwise to formulate a clinical diagnosis of cervicitis without the appropriate microbiological confirmation.

Organisms which cause infections of the female genital tract

Yeasts Yeasts are fungi. *Candida albicans* and *Candida glabrata* are the two most common causes of yeast infection of the vagina, although other Candida species such as *Candida stellatoidea* may well also cause infection. It is important to note that *Candida* occurs as a commensal in the vagina of most women and it is often asymptomatic. The presence of *Candida* on a cervical smear is often an incidental finding and there is no need to provide treatment unless the patient has symptoms.

Symptoms of monilia include the presence of a vaginal discharge and vulval irritation. The vaginal discharge which is associated with *Candida* infection is characteristically described as being a thick caseous white vaginal discharge. However the spectrum is wide and co-existing infections may also be present. *Candida* species may be isolated by culture from a high vaginal swab. When considering treatment for the patient it is important to take note of any predisposing factors that would make the woman more susceptible to infection with *Candida* in the vagina and these include the following:

- Pregnancy
- Use of the combined oral contraceptive pill
- Use of broad-spectrum antibiotics
- Debilitating conditions (e.g. immunodeficient states)
- Diabetes mellitus

The treatment for *Candida* should include simple advice to avoid foods that are rich in sugar and to consume more 'live' yoghurt. The use of fungicides in the form of oral tablets, vaginal ointments or pessaries is usually highly effective.

Trichomonas vaginalis   *Trichomonas vaginalis* (TV) is a motile protozoan with four flagella and an undulating membrane. The organism contains a protrusion shaped like a spike at the opposite end of the four flagella which share a common origin. *Trichomonas vaginalis* infects the vagina and cervix and produces a frothy green irritating vaginal discharge. The patient usually complains of a malodorous copious vaginal discharge associated with severe vulval irritation. Trichomonads may be observed in the cervical smear and may cause inflammatory changes which obscure the accurate cytological reading of cervical smears.

The diagnosis of TV may be reliably made by light microscopic observation of a 'wet' preparation and by isolation by culture from a high vaginal swab. The organism is cultured in the laboratory in the Feinburg–Whittingdon medium. It is advisable to treat the patient's partner(s) as well as the patient herself. The options for treatment include a course of oral metronidazole tablets or a single dose of nimovazole.

Bacterial vaginosis   This has been likened to an 'overgrowth' of anaerobes in the vagina and is a common cause of vaginal discharge. The bacterium *Gardnerella vaginalis* and other anaerobic organisms infect the vagina and large numbers of Gram-negative cocco bacilli may be seen infiltrating around the edges of the vaginal epithelial cells on light microscopic examination of a Gram-stained preparation of a vaginal swab. The appearance of the vaginal epithelial cells with surrounding cocco bacilli is termed the 'clue cell'. There are four diagnostic criteria for a diagnosis of bacterial vaginosis and they are:

1. The presence of 'clue cells'
2. The presence of a malodorous vaginal discharge which is homogenous in consistency
3. A vaginal pH of less than 4.5
4. A positive amine test in which potassium hydroxide is added to a sample of material taken from the vagina and ammonia is released.

At least two of the four diagnostic criteria must be fulfilled before you can establish a diagnosis of bacterial vaginosis. The condition usually responds very well to treatment with amoxicillin or metronidazole tablets taken orally.

Chlamydia trachomatis   *Chlamydia trachomatis* is neither a virus nor a bacterium, although it has properties of both. *Chlamydia psittaci* and *C. trachomatis* share a common genus-specific antigen. *Chlamydia trachomatis* has various different serotypes and they are responsible for three major groups of infections: lymphogranuloma venereum, endemic blinding trachoma and infections of the genital tract in men and women. *Chlamydia trachomatis* may cause cervicitis, salpingitis and acute pelvic inflammatory disease in women, acute urethritis and epididymitis in men and inclusion conjunctivitis and pneumonia in the newborn.

Chlamydial infection of the cervix may be asymptomatic or the patient may complain of a vaginal discharge. *Chlamydia trachomatis* may be identified in endocervical and endourethral swabs taken from patients. If you are taking a swab for *Chlamydia trachomatis* it is mandatory to ask for the patient's permission and to obtain her verbal consent before you do so.

Before inserting an endocervical swab into the cervical canal it is good practice to 'clean' the cervix using a sterile cotton-wool ball. The swab is then inserted into the endocervical canal and gently twisted from side to side for at least 15 seconds.

Chlamydial infection of the cervix may be eradicated with a course of doxycycline or erythromycin tablets. A single dose of oral azithromycin should be adequate to eradicate both chlamydial and gonococcal infection of the cervix but *not* for pelvic inflammatory disease. In practice it is essential to refer a patient with chlamydial infection of the cervix to a specialist in genitourinary medicine. The complications of untreated chlamydial infection of the cervix include acute pelvic inflammatory disease, a predisposition to ectopic pregnancy and salpingitis with perihepatitis. The patient may well become infertile.

Neisseria gonorrhoeae   *Neisseria gonorrhoeae* is a Gram-negative intracellular diplococcus and a well-known sexually transmitted pathogen. The organism infects columnar epithelium (similar sites to *Chlamydia trachomatis*) and these include the lining of the urethra, the cervix and the lining of the Fallopian tubes. It is important to note that *Neisseria gonorrhoeae* does not infect the vagina. Gonococcal infection of the female genital tract may cause vaginal discharge and pelvic pain; the infection may, however, be totally asymptomatic. An asymptomatic woman with gonococcal infection of the cervix is capable of transmitting the disease to a male sexual partner.

Although not as common as chlamydial infection of the cervix it is extremely important to realize that gonorrhoea is still prevalent in the Western world and is rife in many developing countries. Gram-negative intracellular diplococci may be observed on light microscopic examination of a Gram-stained specimen taken from a vaginal swab; however the identification of such an organism on light microscopy does *not* warrant a diagnosis. The laboratory would process any specimens you send and attempt to isolate the organism by culture in Thayer–Martin medium. Following isolation by culture, the laboratory would carry out sugar fermentation tests and immunological identification of the organisms. Provided that all these steps have been taken and the appropriate report has been issued you are now in a position to establish a diagnosis of gonorrhoea. In addition the laboratory may well carry out plasmid determination for epidemiological reasons.

The treatment of gonorrhoea must be left to a specialist in genitourinary medicine. Strains of gonorrhoea which are sensitive to penicillin are best treated by an intramuscular injection of procaine penicillin together with oral probenecid tablets. Strains which are resistant to pencillin (betalactamase-producing organisms) may be treated with either cefuroxime, spectinomycin or augmentin (ampicillin with clavulanic acid). Women with gonorrhoea (even if asymptomatic) are at risk of salpingitis, pelvic inflammatory disease, ectopic pregnancy, perihepatitis and infertility.

Human papilloma virus (HPV)   Human papilloma virus causes genital warts and may also produce abnormalities in cervical smears. The clinical spectrum of disease is wide. The patient may develop a grape-like cluster of warts in the vulva, perineum or vagina. On the other hand the organism may cause nothing other than cytological or histological changes in the cervix. Human papilloma virus types 16 and 18 have been associated with the possible development of invasive cancer of the cervix. Genital warts can be recognized on inspection. Small lesions may be treated by the local application of podophyllin resin every 2–3 days. Such treatment is best provided by specialist doctors and nurses in the genitourinary clinic. Larger lesions require diathermy excision under general anaesthesia in a gynaecological unit.

It is important to note that genital warts grow quickly during pregnancy.

Herpes simplex virus (HSV)   Infection with HSV causes ulceration of mucous membranes. Herpes simplex virus infection of the female genital tract leads to the development of multiple painful genital ulcers. Following an incubation period of 3–4 days the lesions may be located in the vulva, vagina or cervix, producing a considerable level of pain and tenderness for the woman. Syphilitic ulcers on the other hand produce solitary painless ulcers and chancroid (produced by *Haemophilus ducreyi*) produces large multiple painful ulcers. Infection with HSV is one of the most common causes of genital ulcers in both women and men.

Herpes simplex virus may be isolated by culture from swabs taken from lesions. The organism may also be identified using electron microscopy in preparations obtained from the lesions. An asymptomatic woman may well shed the virus into the vaginal secretions. The typical pattern of genital infection with HSV follows a severe initial attack followed by spontaneous resolution and recurrent attacks (even in the absence of sexual activity) which lead to further ulcers and symptoms. The recurrent attacks tend to decrease in severity, duration and frequency of occurrence.

Herpes simplex virus infections may be treated with aciclovir topical cream and aciclovir tablets; however, some types of HSV are resistant to aciclovir, and other options currently available include either famciclovir or valaciclovir tablets. A woman with HSV infection of the lower genital tract is best referred to a physician practising genitourinary medicine. If the patient is also pregnant you will need to alert the consultant obstetrician who is sharing her care with you.

Hepatitis B virus   Although hepatitis B virus does not cause any lesions in the lower female genital tract it is important to recognize that the hepatitis B virus (HBV) may be transmitted parenterally, sexually and perinatally. The majority of patients with HBV infection resolve the infection spontaneously and develop natural immunity. However it is essential to realize that rare complications of HBV infection include acute liver failure, chronic hepatitis (with its consequences) and liver cancer.

As a generalization it is important to note that sexually transmitted (or transmissible) pathogens 'hunt in pairs and packs'. If you have diagnosed the presence of sexually transmitted disease in a patient you should consider testing for HBV infection. If the patient has HBV infection she should be counselled appropriately and her liver function must be investigated. The newborn may be protected against transmission of HBV from the mother by a vaccine against the virus (see p.199).

Human immunodeficiency virus   Human immunodeficiency virus (HIV) will ultimately lead to the development of acquired immunodeficiency syndrome (AIDS). Whether or not to test for evidence of HIV infection in a patient depends upon the facilities that are available for counselling, your clinical index for suspicion and epidemiological intelligence on local rates of prevalence. As in all aspects of medical care if you are testing for evidence of HIV infection you must obtain the patient's permission to do so and confidentiality must be maintained.

Special situations

Antenatal care in a woman with infection of the genital tract   If you are aware that a woman has a sexually transmitted disease and she reports for antenatal care you must ask for her consent to relay that information to the professionals in obstetrics and midwifery who are sharing her care with you. Some infections such as syphilis can lead to early pregnancy as well as late pregnancy loss. If it is left untreated syphilis may produce a significant level of mental and physical handicap during childhood and indeed in later years. There is some evidence that untreated chlamydial infection of the cervix may lead to ruptured membranes and pre-term labour. The patient with large genital warts during pregnancy may require diathermy excision of the lesions under general anaesthesia.

Infection of the genital tract in a woman undergoing termination of pregnancy   There is evidence that untreated cervical and gonococcal infection of the cervix predisposes a woman to developing post-abortal pelvic inflammatory disease. Patients who are in this situation must be given the appropriate pre-operative counselling and treatment.

Vestibulitis   Patients with vestibulitis complain of discomfort following sexual intercourse, vulval irritation and a burning vaginal discharge. The pain may extend into the perineum and natal cleft. It is debatable as to whether or not the vestibulitis is due to an infectious inflammation. In any case patients with vulvodynia may represent a difficult problem in management for general practitioners and indeed specialists as the swabs which are taken are invariably 'negative'. Patients with vestibulitis often do not have any clinical signs either. Options for treatment include the use of an emulsifying ointment as a substitute for soap and 5% lidocaine (lignocaine) ointment applied topically to the vulva and perineum. If these measures fail to work over a 3-week period amitriptyline at a low starting dosage is an alternative option for the control of pain. If the treatment with amitriptyline is also unsuccessful you must refer the patient to a pain clinic. Although patients with the symptoms of vestibulitis may well have stressful jobs and lives the condition is nevertheless well described and it is important to acknowledge the patient's symptoms.

Pelvic inflammatory disease (PID) A patient with pelvic inflammatory disease will experience lower abdominal pain, vaginal discharge, dyspareunia and may well be febrile. The important differential diagnoses include unruptured ectopic pregnancy, the early stages of acute appendicitis and acute pyelonephritis.

Box 4.5   Pelvic inflammatory disease

Aetiology   Polymicrobial – several different organisms including *Chlamydia trachomatis, Neisseria gonorrhoeae* and anaerobes have been implicated as causes of acute pelvic inflammatory disease in women. The fact that different organisms may well be involved in a single episode requires the use of broad-spectrum antibiotic coverage when considering treatment.

Pathogenesis   The patient develops salpingitis and then salpingo-oophoritis as a result of ascending infection from the lower genital tract. The Fallopian tubes become swollen, inflamed and a purulent exudate is released into the peritoneal cavity. Inflammatory adhesions form and a pelvic abscess may well develop. The patient may develop pelvic peritonitis and parts of the bowel may become tethered to infected sites in the pelvis.

Symptoms   The main symptoms of acute pelvic inflammatory disease are lower abdominal pain, vaginal discharge, dyspareunia, dysuria, a feeling of being unwell and raised temperature.

Signs   Lower abdominal tenderness and pelvic tenderness on bimanual palpation. The vagina characteristically feels warm or 'hot' when the examining finger is inserted into the organ. Cervical excitation is usually present. In advanced cases the patient may well have an adnexal mass which is a purulent tubo-ovarian collection.

Investigation   The presence of fever, neutrophil leucocytosis and 'positive' swabs serve to complete the picture of pelvic inflammatory disease but it is important to note that none of these may be present. The patient's temperature may well be normal in cases of chlamydial pelvic inflammatory disease and the white cell count may also be normal. In addition, the failure to recover organisms from swabs of the lower genital tract does not exclude the presence of salpingo-oophoritis or a pelvic abscess involving the upper genital tract.

Treatment   Patients with a febrile pelvic inflammatory disease with pain should be admitted to the acute gynaecology ward and treated with intravenous antibiotics. In many cases the general practitioner may feel able to treat the patient on an outpatient basis and it is essential to prescribe antibiotics which will eradicate the organisms which may well be involved in the pathogenesis of the disease. Standard regimens for treatment using oral antibiotics include the following:

- Doxycycline 100 mg twice daily for 15 days together with metronidazole 400 mg thrice daily for 7 days
- Erythromycin 500 mg four times daily for 10 days together with metronidazole 400 mg thrice daily for 7 days

The response to treatment with antibiotics is usually rapid – within 24–48 hours the patient's condition improves considerably. From the point of view of the specialist, surgery may be required under the following circumstances:

1. Diagnostic laparoscopy in order to establish a diagnosis of pelvic inflammatory disease and to exclude other conditions such as ectopic pregnancy.
2. Laparotomy for a patient with a ruptured abscess and pelvic peritonitis.
3. Laparotomy in order to drain an expanding pelvic abscess which has failed to respond to parenteral antibiotics.

A patient with febrile illness and a significant level of tenderness on pelvic examination must be referred to a specialist on an urgent basis. Patients with signs of pelvic peritonitis and ruptured pelvic abscess must be referred to a specialist on an emergency basis.

Summary of investigations   It is difficult to perform a comprehensive list of investigations on each and every patient. You may however find the following list to be a useful summary:

- Endourethral swab – *Chlamydia trachomatis*, *Neisseria gonorrhoeae*
- Endocervical swab – *Chlamydia trachomatis*, *Neisseria gonorrhoeae*
- High vaginal swab – *Candida*, *Trichomonas vaginalis*, evidence for

bacterial vaginosis, bacterial culture and sensitivity tests
- Rectal swab – *Neisseria gonorrhoeae*
- Vulval swab – herpes simplex virus
- Serology – syphilis, HIV, HBV

INFERTILITY

Approximately 10% of couples experience infertility and a significant number of patients see their GP concerning the problem. A healthy heterosexual couple who have regular coitus (approximately twice per week) should achieve pregnancy within one year. Over 50% of such couples achieve pregnancy after 6 cycles and over 90% by the end of 12 cycles. In practice infertility is defined as the inability of a heterosexual couple to achieve pregnancy after 12 months of trying to do so. Infertility may be associated with both male and female factors and the GP has a pivotal role to play in the overall management of infertile couples.

Causes
A significant proportion of couples with infertility have 'idiopathic' infertility where no cause for the condition is determined. Some conditions such as pelvic endometriosis are associated with infertility even if the Fallopian tubes are patent. The following conditions either cause or are associated with infertility:

- Azospermia
- Oligospermia with defective spermatozoa
- Problems with coitus
- Infrequent coitus
- Anovulation
- Cervical mucus hostility
- Bilateral tubal occlusive disease
- Idiopathic

Management
The Royal College of Obstetricians and Gynaecologists has issued evidence-based guidelines for the management of infertility both in primary and secondary care. It is important to develop local protocols based on these guidelines and to adhere to them. The general practitioner should take an adequate and appropriate history from the infertile couple. Such a history would include the standard gynaecological history (see p. 86) together with details of frequency of sexual intercourse, whether or not adequate penetration occurs and a detailed history of any previous pregnancies. The male partner should be asked about a history of diseases of the genital tract including sexually transmitted disease, previous illnesses and whether or not he already has children by a previous partner. An occupational history from

both partners is essential as environmental factors can play a significant role in fertility. Couples should be advised to have regular coitus throughout the cycle. Box 4.6 lists further advice a GP should give a couple trying to conceive.

There is no evidence to support the use of basal body temperature charts as a means of providing a guide to timed sexual intercourse around about the time of ovulation. It is important to realize that infertile couples are often highly anxious and they must be encouraged to relax and not feel under pressure.

The GP should arrange investigations in order to determine whether or not the patient is ovulating by measuring the mid-luteal serum progesterone. Basically the woman's serum progesterone is measured 7 days prior to the expected start of her next period. If she has irregular menstrual cycles then the serum TSH and prolactin levels should be measured. A mid-luteal serum progesterone in excess of 30 nmol/l is proof of adequate ovulation in a particular cycle.

The male partner should have two semen analyses. It is useful to determine what your local laboratory's parameters are for a 'normal' semen

---

Box 4.6   Practical advice for patients experiencing infertility

1. Women with infertility should be strongly urged to stop smoking cigarettes. Similar advice should also be offered to the male partner.
2. Alcohol intake should be limited to 1–2 units of alcohol once or twice a week.
3. If the woman is seronegative for rubella then rubella vaccination should be offered and the patient advised not to become pregnant within 1 month of vaccination.
4. Women experiencing infertility should be advised to take 0.4 mg folic acid orally every day while they are trying to conceive and to continue during the first 12 weeks of a pregnancy. In the case of women with a previous history of having had a child with a neural tube defect or those receiving anti-convulsant treatment the dosage of folic acid should be 5 mg orally once a day.
5. If the patient's body mass index (weight divided by height squared) is greater than 30 then she should be asked to join a weight-reduction programme.
6. The GP should review medications which may affect ovulation. For example, the following cause hyperprolactinaemia:

   • Tricyclic anti-depressants
   • Phenothiazines
   • Monoamine oxidase inhibitors
   • Metoclopramide
   • Alphamethyldopa

---

analysis but the following values, reproduced from the World Health Organization (WHO), provide some guidance.

- Volume: 2–5 ml
- Liquefaction time: within 30 min
- Concentration: more than 20 million spermatozoa per ml
- Motility: more than 50% progressive motility
- Morphology: more than 30% normal forms
- White blood cells: less than 1 million/ml

Patients should be referred appropriately to a specialist infertility unit if one is available. Female patients with the following should be considered for early referral:

1. Age in excess of 35 years
2. Amenorrhoea
3. Oligomenorrhoea
4. Previous abdominal or pelvic surgery
5. Previous history of pelvic inflammatory disease or sexually transmitted disease
6. Abnormalities on pelvic examination

Further investigations
A GP would not be involved in the further investigations and specialist treatment of causes of infertility; it is however important to know what your patients are likely to undergo after they have been seen by a specialist. In a specialist service it is standard policy to complete the initial investigations and advice given to patients. Following that the specialists would advise the patient to undergo a laparoscopy and dye test to provide the following information:

- Appearance of the uterus, Fallopian tubes and ovaries
- Patency of the Fallopian tubes
- Cause (if present) of tubal occlusive disease
- Presence (at the appropriate time in the cycle) of corpus luteum in either ovary
- Presence of pelvic endometriosis, adhesions or sepsis
- To study the accessibility of the ovaries in case assisted reproduction needs to be considered at a later date.

In addition, the specialist may arrange for a more detailed endocrine profile of the patient.

Treatment
The treatment of any condition depends on the underlying cause.
Anovulation may be treated using clomifene which is given as an oral dose between day 2 to day 6 (inclusive). It is important to note that clomifene may lead to the formation of ovarian cysts, to multiple pregnancy and it can

also cause diplopia in a minority of patients, although diplopia is reversed once the patient stops taking clomifene. If you prescribe the drug to a patient it is important to advise her of the side effects and arrange measurement of the mid-luteal serum progesterone in order to determine whether ovulation is taking place, as well as pelvic and ultrasound examination at regular intervals in order to detect the formation of ovarian cysts.

No patient should be given clomifene for more than 6 cycles consecutively. The initial daily dosage is 50 mg to be taken as previously described. The dosage can subsequently be increased to 100 mg and then 150 mg.

More sophisticated techniques for induction of ovulation are best left to a specialist infertility unit (see p. 115).

Patients with anovulation secondary to hyperprolactinaemia should be treated with a dopamine agonist such as cabergoline (dosage 0.5 mg to 1.0 mg orally once a week) or bromocriptine (2.5 mg orally twice daily). Patients with hyperprolactinaemia would also need to undergo the appropriate pituitary imaging either by magnetic resonance imaging (MRI) or by computerized axial tomography (CAT) which a specialist would arrange.

The current approach to patients with bilateral tubal occlusive disease is to consider referral for in vitro fertilization (see p. 115). Few centres in the UK practice tubal surgery which requires the use of the appropriately trained staff, microsurgical techniques and specialist counselling.

ASSISTED REPRODUCTION

Some patients require the use of sophisticated surgical or mechanical techniques to achieve fertilization and/or transfer of an embryo to the uterus. In most cases the couple's own gametes are used. However it is important to note that spermatozoa or oocytes may be donated. Some couples enter into private arrangements for surrogate pregnancy. In 1984 the Warnock Report produced a set of recommendations that have influenced policy in assisted reproduction. It is important to note that centres practising in vitro fertilization, embryo transfer, embryo freezing and research on embryos must have the appropriate licence.

Counselling

Patients who undergo assisted reproduction receive appropriate counselling from the specialist (or sub-specialist) who takes responsibility for the treatment. A GP must understand the following:

- The nature of the procedure to be used.
- The fact that any procedure that involves induction of ovulation by serial injections of gonadotrophins literally 'takes over' the couple's life, as the patient needs to be at certain places at certain times throughout the cycle.
- There is a risk of ovarian hyperstimulation if induction of ovulation is being carried out.

- The success rate in terms of a term pregnancy varies from procedure to procedure and from centre to centre and is influenced by the age of the female partner. For example the success rate following in vitro fertilization and embryo transfer is approximately 1/6 for a woman who is less than 35 years old, falling to 1/20 for a woman who is aged 40.
- There is a risk of multiple pregnancy following the induction of ovulation.
- Disorders of implantation may prevent pregnancy following successful in vitro fertilization or embryo transfer (IVF) or successful gamete intra-Fallopian transfer (GIFT).

Induction of ovulation with intrauterine insemination

Following the initial visit and counselling the patient receives hormonal treatment (usually with GnRH analogues) to down-regulate her menstrual cycle. Following this the patient is given serial injections of human menopausal gonadotrophin (FSH) with an appropriately timed injection of human chorionic gonadotrophin to mimic the physiological action of LH. The time of ovulation can therefore be predicted with a high level of accuracy and the patient undergoes either artificial insemination using her partner's semen (AIH) or artificial insemination using donor semen (AID). Semen donors undergo extensive screening for infections and genetic disorders; the patient would also have received detailed counselling from the licensed sub-specialist centre prior to AID.

Prior to induction of ovulation and artificial insemination it is essential to establish that the patient's Fallopian tubes are patent (see p. 147). For an otherwise healthy woman with patent Fallopian tubes whose partner has normal semen analysis the success rate, in terms of a term pregnancy, following induction of ovulation and AIH and AID is in the order of 1/6.

In vitro fertilization and embryo transfer

In practice this particular procedure takes place in sub-specialist centres. Detailed counselling is necessary prior to IVF. The procedure involves sedation but a general anaesthetic is rarely required. The indications for IVF and embryo transfer are as follows:

- Oligospermia
- Bilateral tubal occlusive disease
- Anovulatory disorders
- Idiopathic infertility

The patient undergoes induction of ovulation and pre-ovulatory ovarian follicles are retrieved by ultrasound guided needle aspiration of the ovaries. The oocytes are incubated with prepared semen from the patient's partner and a maximum of three embryos are transferred to the patient's uterus. There is no evidence of an association between in vitro fertilization and fetal abnormality.

Gamete intra-Fallopian transfer

GIFT may be performed either in sub-specialist centres or in a district general hospital but it is important to have an appropriately trained team. The patient undergoes induction of ovulation and egg collection as described in the previous section. Semen from the partner is collected and prepared appropriately. The prepared semen and up to three eggs are introduced (together) into the fimbrial end of the Fallopian tube. The objective of the procedure is to enable fertilization within the Fallopian tube and natural implantation. It is important to note that GIFT involves the use of laparoscopy under general anaesthesia.

There is no evidence of an association between GIFT and fetal abnormality. However it is important to note that both IVF and GIFT are associated with an increased risk of ectopic pregnancy.

COLPOSCOPY

Cervical cytology, colposcopy and histopathology of the cervix variously answer three very different questions.

- Cervical cytology answers the question 'Is there a problem?'
- Colposcopy answers the question 'Where (in the cervix or vagina) is the problem?'
- Histopathology answers the question 'What exactly is the problem?'

The United Kingdom has a national cervical screening programme for women with a recall system and ready access to colposcopy services. General practitioners perform a key role in the supervision of screening for pre-malignant disease of the cervix by cervical cytology and referral of appropriate patients for further investigations.

Cervical cytology

It is essential that you are able to perform a pelvic examination, pass a Cusco speculum and take an adequate smear. Patients should undergo regular cervical smear tests between the ages of 20 and 65 years, with an interval of 5 years in between normal cervical smears. The following factors place a woman at risk of developing pre-malignant disease of the cervix:

- Low age at first coitus
- Multiple sexual partners
- History of sexually transmitted disease, especially genital wart virus infection
- Immunosuppression

The cytologist who examines the smear decides whether it is normal or abnormal and assesses the degree of cervical dysplasia. Cytological criteria include the shape and size of the cells, the thickness of the cell membrane, the appearance of the cytoplasm, the morphological appearance of the nucleus, the number and appearance of mitoses and the ratio of the size of the nucleus to the amount of cytoplasm in the same cell. The result of a cervical smear may be any one of the following:

- Normal (negative)
- Inflammatory
- Inadequate for assessment
- Borderline
- Mild dysplasia
- Moderate dysplasia
- Severe dysplasia
- ?Microinvasive disease
- ?Invasive cancer of the cervix
- Glandular atypia
- ?Adenocarcinoma

An inflammatory appearance in the cervical smear may be due to the presence of untreated infection of the cervix. The infection may well be sexually transmitted (see p. 105) and the appropriate investigations and treatment would then be necessary. On occasions the cytologist is able to detect specific infections such as *Candida* or *Trichomonas vaginalis*.

The following simple rules help to plan the management of patients with an abnormal cervical smear.

1. Severe dyskaryosis? invasive carcinoma – refer on an urgent basis to a gynaecological oncologist.
2. Glandular neoplasia – refer urgently to a gynaecological oncologist
3. Severe dyskaryosis – refer for colposcopy
4. Moderate dyskaryosis – refer for colposcopy
5. Mild dyskaryosis on two occasions – refer for colposcopy
6. Borderline result on two or three occasions – refer for colposcopy

It is helpful to remember that cervical smears are carried out to screen for pre-malignant disease of the cervix. A cervical smear may be 'negative' in the presence of an invasive carcinoma of the cervix and every healthcare worker who carries out cervical smears should inspect the cervix carefully prior to taking a cervical smear.

Colposcopic examination
Colposcopic examination of the vulva, vagina and cervix must be carried out by a doctor who has been appropriately trained to the standards of the British Society of Colposcopy and Cervical Pathology. Colposcopy consists of examining a specific object (cervix, vagina or vulva) using a system of optical magnification. The cervix is inspected without any preparation apart from cleaning with sterile saline solution, after application of acetic acid and of Lugol's iodine. The colposcopist looks for the squamo-columnar junction, variations in structure of the connective tissue and the underlying vascularity,

together with physiological and pathological changes. Overt lesions may also be identified during a colposcopic examination of the cervix.

The purpose of colposcopy is to identify the presence and position of lesions in the cervix. As a general practitioner you would not need to know the technical details but it is important for you to be able to explain to patients exactly what the procedure entails. Colposcopic examination of the cervix may well be accompanied by treatment of pre-malignant lesions of the cervix.

You must be able to convey the information in Box 4.7 to the patient whom you are referring for a colposcopic examination of the cervix +/- local treatment to the cervix.

For various reasons a colposcopic examination of the cervix may not be feasible or it may be inconclusive. Under such circumstances the specialist may well recommend a cone biopsy of the cervix under general anaesthesia.

Treatment

Following the diagnosis of cervical intraepithelial neoplasia the lesion may either be destroyed or excised. Examples of destructive therapy include:

- Carbon dioxide laser ablation
- Cryosurgery
- Cold coagulation
- Electrocoagulation

Box 4.7   Information for a patient referred for colposcopic examination

1. The procedure involves an 'internal' examination.
2. A brief description of the method, including the need for staining the cervix.
3. The procedure takes approximately 5–10 minutes without any treatment and up to 15 minutes with treatment.
4. Local anaesthesia is provided as an injection into the cervix (rather than, for example, the forearm).
5. The nature of any treatment.
6. Local treatment of the cervix does not affect cervical function or the patient's obstetric future.
7. The patient may well experience uterine contractions leading to cramp-like lower abdominal pain during treatment.
8. The treatment is highly successful in most cases.
9. Follow-up is required.
10. Possible complications include bleeding and infection.
11. The most common aftermath of treatment is a bloodstained vaginal discharge which may take over 2 weeks to resolve.
12. The colposcopy clinic provides the patient with a means of seeking urgent attention should it be necessary to do so following treatment.

Examples of methods of excision include:

- Large loop excision of the transformation zone (LLETZ) usually under local anaesthesia
- Cone biopsy using a scalpel under general anaesthesia
- Cone biopsy using laser under general anaesthesia

In the management of some patients a hysterectomy may well be required.

Histopathology

The pathologist will identify the exact nature of the lesion. Pre-malignant disease of the cervix is graded as cervical intraepithelial neoplasia (CIN) I, II or III depending on the severity. CIN III is far more likely to progress to invasive carcinoma of the cervix than CIN I. 'Microinvasive' carcinoma of the cervix is a specific histological diagnosis which is established after examining a sizeable piece of tissue; in practice a cone biopsy or a 'wedge' biopsy. Invasive carcinoma of the cervix is a malignant lesion of the cervix with a significant risk of involvement of the pelvic lymph nodes.

Follow-up

It is essential to carry out the appropriate follow-up for patients who have undergone treatment for pre-malignant lesions of the cervix. Patients who have had treatment may have residual disease, they may develop new disease or they may even develop invasive cancer of the cervix. Following local treatment to the cervix for CIN II or CIN III the protocol outlined in Box 4.8 (or one very similar to it) would be used by most units.

Box 4.8   Protocol following treatment for CIN II or CIN III

1. Cervical smear +/- colposcopic examination of the cervix 4 months following treatment.
2. If the cervical smear is negative, repeat a cervical smear (without colposcopy) 12 months later.
3. If the second cervical smear is negative repeat a cervical smear annually for 4 years.
4. If all the cervical smears are negative carry out screening with cervical smears every 3 years.

If the patient has undergone hysterectomy for CIN II or CIN III carry out vaginal vault smears at 6 and 12 months post-operatively. If both the cervical smears are negative then further follow-up may be discontinued. However, if there is any doubt whatsoever that the pre-malignant lesion has not been removed completely it would be advisable to seek the help of a specialist. If the patient has undergone hysterectomy for benign disease of the genital tract and histological examination of the cervix shows no abnormality then there is no need to carry out any vault smears.

VULVAL DISEASES

Diseases of the vulva may present with pruritus vulvae, vulval pain and soreness, the presence of a lump – or they may be totally asymptomatic. The GP may detect the presence of a lesion on the vulva by careful inspection during the course of a pelvic examination.

Causes of pruritus vulvae

Pruritus vulvae may be caused by infections in the vagina such as *Trichomonas vaginalis*, bacterial vaginosis or moniliasis. It is important to note, however, that various vulval diseases may also cause pruritus vulvae. It is a common diagnostic pitfall to carry out various investigations for the detection of a vaginal condition as a cause of pruritus vulvae when the actual cause may well be a condition of the vulval epithelium. In addition tinea cruris of the groins and pediculosis pubis infestation may occasionally be mistaken for 'pruritus vulvae'.

The following vulval diseases may cause pruritus vulvae:

- Lichen sclerosus et atrophicus
- Vulval intraepithelial neoplasia (VIN)
- Vulval warts
- Vulval cancer
- Vulval melanoma
- Vulval hydradenitis suppuritiva
- Psoriasis
- Eczema
- Allergic dermatitis
- Paget's disease.

Clinical management

The general practitioner should refer women with vulval diseases to the appropriate specialist for further investigations and management. Several of the conditions that have been listed in the previous section require histological diagnosis and grading. A specialist would arrange vulval biopsy under local or general anaesthesia depending on the individual clinical circumstances. Furthermore the treatment of several of the conditions is far from perfect and the supervision of a specialist is appropriate. In the absence of an obvious lesion the diagnosis of vulvodynia must be considered (see p. 110).

Lichen sclerosus

This is the equivalent lesion in women of balanitis xerotica obliterans in men. The disease and its treatment are outlined in Box 4.9.

Vulval intraepithelial neoplasia

VIN is the equivalent in the vulva of CIN in the cervix. Vulval intraepithelial neoplasia is a disease in which neoplastic cells are contained within the boundaries of the surface epithelium. The diagnosis and grading of VIN are based on histological examination of a biopsy sample. The disease and its treatment are outlined in Box 4.10.

Box 4.9   Lichen sclerosus

Symptoms	Superficial dyspareunia Delayed vulval healing (for example following episiotomy) Pruritus vulvae
Clinical signs	White and thin vulval skin Affected areas include the labia, clitoris, perineum and perianal area producing a 'dumb-bell'-shaped lesion Fusion of the labia minora Narrowing of the introitus
Diagnosis	Vulval biopsy and histological examination
Treatment	Topical corticosteroids
Risk of progression to vulval carcinoma	Less than 5%

Box 4.10   Vulval intraepithelial neoplasia

Symptoms	Pruritus vulvae Vulval soreness Asymptomatic The presence of a lump (rare)
Clinical signs	Papular and coarse lesions which may appear like genital warts Lesions which appear macular with irregular borders Hyperkeratosis Ulceration Pigmentation (brown/black) Colposcopically detectable following the application of 2% acetic acid to the vulva
Treatment options include:	Excision biopsy Vulvectomy Topical 5-fluorouracil Topical dinitrochlorobenzene Cryosurgery Carbon dioxide laser ablation Topical alpha interferon gel
Risk of progression to vulval cancer	Approximately 8%

Risk factors for progression to vulval carcinoma	Presentation in the post-menopausal age group Unifocal, rather than multifocal, lesion Excessive hyperkeratosis Immune deficiency Histologically progressive lesions as seen on serial vulval biopsy

PELVIC MASS

GPs commonly see patients with a pelvic mass: the investigation and clinical management of each case is dependent on the patient's clinical circumstances. The following simple steps will assist you in determining the underlying cause for a pelvic mass.

- An adequate case history including symptoms of pregnancy, weight gain, weight loss; history of abdominal or pelvic pain; cyclical nature of the symptoms; urinary symptoms; gastrointestinal symptoms.
- Physical examination including speculum, vaginal and possibly a rectal examination of the pelvis
- Urinary pregnancy test
- Full blood count
- An appropriate form of pelvic imaging
- Serum tumour marker levels

The GP would be able to request an ultrasound examination of the pelvis in most centres but more sophisticated requests for computerized axial tomography or magnetic resonance imaging would need to come from a specialist. Serum tumours markers include serum Ca 125 for tumours of ovarian epithelial origin, serum beta HCG for pregnancy and (non-gestational) trophoblastic tumours and serum alpha fetoprotein for endodermal sinus tumour.

Causes
The following may be the causes of a pelvic mass.

- Full bladder
- Full rectum
- Gravid uterus
- Uterine fibroids
- Uterine leiomyosarcoma
- Ovarian cyst
- Ovarian tumour

- Ectopic pregnancy
- Hydrosalpinx
- Endometriosis
- Haematocolpos
- Pelvic kidney
- Carcinoma of the bowel
- Massive faecal impaction
- Abscess related to diverticular disease
- Abscess related to inflammatory bowel disease

OVARIAN CYSTS

Benign functional cysts of the ovary are the most common manifestation of an ovarian cyst. Polycystic ovarian syndrome can lead to the development of mild ovarian enlargement with multiple small cysts located in the periphery of each ovary. It is important, however, to note that no other organ in the human body can lead to the development of such a diverse range of tumours. The ovaries may also be a site for secondary spread from malignant tumours at other sites.

Pathology
Ovarian tumours are difficult to classify for various reasons. The cause is largely unknown, the histopathological picture may be confusing, different types of tumour may co-exist in the same lesion and the hormonal effects of endocrinologically active tumours may be variable. An ovarian cyst may be physiological or pathological. Pathological lesions may be unilateral or bilateral, cystic or solid. A cystic ovarian tumour may be unilocular or multi-locular. Pathological enlargement of the ovary may be the result of a benign or malignant lesion.

The following classification is simplified but useful for the GP. Ovarian tumours are considered to arise from any one or more of the cell layers which constitute the embryological origin of the ovary. The ovary consists of ectodermal cells from the coelomic epithelium, stromal cells within the mesenchyme underlying the coelomic epithelium and endodermal cells. Endodermal cells migrate from the embryonic yolk sac and give rise to the eggs in the ovary. Therefore, any or all of these three basic cell layers may lead to ovarian tumours. Using this concept ovarian tumours may be classified as follows.

1. Tumours arising from the epithelium – examples include tumours of epithelial origin such as the benign serous or mucinous cystadenoma and

malignant tumours such as the serous cystadenocarcinoma or mucinous cystadenocarcinoma.   *Oelmogen producing*

2. Tumours of stromal cell origin – examples include the endocrinologically active tumours such as the granulosa cell tumour, theca cell tumour and arrhenoblastoma. *(androgen secreting)*
3. Tumours of germ cell origin – examples include dysgerminoma and endodermal sinus tumour. *+ teratoma*

Serum Ca 125 is associated with ovarian tumours of epithelial origin (see p. 123) and is measured in patients who are suspected of suffering from ovarian cancer or who have undergone treatment for it. Granulosa cell tumours and theca cell tumours produce oestrogen whereas the arrhenoblastoma produces androgens. The endodermal sinus tumour (very rare) secretes alpha fetoprotein. The dermoid cyst, more appropriately termed benign cystic teratoma, contains tissue from all three cell *layers*. A dermoid cyst may contain hair, skin, sebaceous and sweat glands (ectoderm), bone and cartilage (mesoderm) and intestinal mucosa and thyroid epithelium (endoderm).

Complications
A benign ovarian tumour may give rise to the following complications.

- Torsion
- Infection
- Haemorrhage
- Rupture
- Malignant change

A malignant ovarian tumour invades adjacent organs such as the uterus, Fallopian tubes, bladder and rectum, leading to the development of ascites which may be massive and spread intraperitoneally.

Clinical features
A patient who has an ovarian cyst may be totally asymptomatic. However you must consider the possibility of an ovarian cyst in a woman who complains of the following symptoms.

- Pelvic discomfort
- Abdominal distension
- Pain
- Increased frequency of micturition
- Urgency of micturition
- Acute retention of urine (following impaction of the lesion in the pelvis)
- Dyspnoea (large tumours)
- Dyspepsia (large tumours possibly with ascites)

Physical examination of the patient's abdomen and pelvis may well raise the clinical suspicion of an ovarian cyst. Ultrasound examination of the pelvis is invaluable. A specialist would be able to organize more sophisticated forms of imaging (see p. 122).

Management

It is important to remember that the exact diagnosis is often established only after a surgical procedure and histological examination of the lesion. Even then a specialist in pathology may need to seek the opinion of a regional specialist. The histopathological appearance of ovarian lesions can be perplexing. Not all ovarian cysts need to be removed. The decision as to whether or not to intervene surgically is best left to a specialist. Issues which would be taken into account include the risk of malignancy, the severity of symptoms and of course the patient's own wishes.

A small benign ovarian cyst may well be drained at laparoscopy. Larger but benign lesions may be managed by performing laparotomy and ovarian cystectomy or unilateral oophorectomy. If the patient is suspected of having a malignant ovarian lesion then major surgery is indicated (see p. 144)

Special situations

Ovarian cysts complicating pregnancy If an ovarian cyst is detected during pregnancy and the lesion is more than 10 cm in diameter (approximately) then laparotomy and ovarian cystectomy should be considered at 14–16 weeks' gestation. If the tumour is left *in situ* there is an increased risk of torsion, rupture and haemorrhage in later pregnancy. Such a lesion is best managed conservatively during the first trimester so as not to disturb the early pregnancy. Beyond the second trimester of pregnancy surgical access may be problematic.

Borderline tumours Following removal of an ovarian tumour the pathologist may report that the lesion was 'borderline'. A patient with a history of 'borderline' ovarian tumour *must* be registered with a specialist who would then carry out the appropriate follow-up on a long-term basis. Once the patient has completed her family the option of total abdominal hysterectomy and removal of all remaining ovarian tissue may be considered.

Theca lutein cysts of the ovary Theca lutein cysts of the ovary may be quite large, bilateral and they occur in association with a hydatidiform mole. Following the removal of trophoblastic tumour tissue from the patient theca lutein cysts of the ovary resolve spontaneously.

Krukenberg's tumour These rare tumours consist of bilateral, smooth, encapsulated tumours of moderate size. The lesions are produced by secondary deposits from a primary malignancy in the gastrointestinal tract.

Ovarian fibroma These are rare benign tumours which occur in the ovary and are often associated with ascites. Meig's syndrome consists of ovarian fibroma, ascites and pleural effusion. Following removal of the ovarian fibroma the ascites and pleural effusion resolve spontaneously. Although ovarian fibroma is a rare example of an ovarian tumour it is important to remember that ascites due to an ovarian cause may be benign.

PELVIC ENDOMETRIOSIS

The occurrence of endometrium in sites other than the lining of the uterine cavity is referred to as endometriosis. Endometriosis usually occurs in the pelvis although it is important to note that the condition has been described as occurring in the lungs, diaphragm, central nervous system, kidney and surgical scars. More commonly endometriosis occurs in the myometrium of the uterus and this particular condition is termed adenomyosis. The condition affects women in their reproductive years and regresses after the menopause. The condition is common and the GP should be aware of its clinical features, the need for appropriate referral and the options for treatment.

Pathology

The cause of endometriosis is unknown. There may be several mechanisms whereby endometrium starts to develop in ectopic sites. The theories for the aetiology of endometriosis include growth and cyclical bleeding of endometrium from embryonic deposits within the coelomic cavity, retrograde menstruation, and lymphatic and vascular dissemination from the uterine cavity. The ovaries are the most common site for endometriosis and recurrent bleeding may lead to the formation of a 'chocolate cyst' which contains old blood. Other sites for endometriotic deposits include:

- Pelvic peritoneum – especially the rectovaginal septum and the vesicouterine fold of peritoneum.
- Uterosacral ligaments
- Pouch of Douglas
- Round ligaments

The size of endometriotic deposits varies significantly. It is important to note, however, that size may not necessarily correspond with symptoms. A small deposit which is less than 0.5 cm in diameter in the uterosacral ligament could produce more troublesome symptoms for the patient than a large unruptured ovarian chocolate cyst. Endometriosis tissue bleeds in response to the hormones that control the menstrual cycle. Over a period of time adhesions may well develop within the pelvis and the patient occasionally develops what is termed a 'frozen pelvis'.

Clinical features

The symptoms of endometriosis are usually cyclical in nature; they may, however, be very varied and some patients may be asymptomatic. Common symptoms of endometriosis include:

- Dyspareunia
- Dysmenorrhoea
- Menorrhagia
- Infertility
- Pelvic pain
- Pain on defaecation

Rarely patients may present with intermittent haematuria, intermittent fever and symptoms and signs of intestinal obstruction.

The following clinical signs may be found on examination:

- Tender palpable nodules in the pelvis
- Adnexal mass
- Pelvic mass
- Fixed retroverted uterus

Patients with adenomyosis commonly complain of dysmenorrhoea and menorrhagia. On examination they would have a slightly enlarged, tender but mobile uterus.

Diagnosis

Endometriosis must be visualized before the diagnosis is established. In practice this entails referral to a specialist who will carry out gynaecological laparoscopy in order to determine the diagnosis. The diagnosis of endometriosis may also be established at laparotomy and direct inspection. Ultrasound examination of the pelvis is a useful adjunct in the investigation of patients with suspected endometriosis and adenomyosis has a discrete ultrasonic appearance.

Treatment

The treatment of pelvic endometriosis depends on various factors and what is appropriate for one particular patient may be wholly inappropriate for another. The following factors influence the choice of treatment:

1. The age of the patient
2. The patient's views on her own fertility
3. The extent of the symptoms
4. The extent of the disease

It is important to remember that endometriosis does not become malignant and it does tend to regress following the menopause. As a GP you would be involved in the appropriate referral of patients for specialist investigation and treatment. The general practitioner may use hormonal forms of treatment such as the combined oral contraceptive pill given continuously for 6 months or oral medroxyprogesterone acetate given continuously for the same period. Other forms of treatment should be left to the supervision of a specialist. Box 4.11 is a summary of options for treatment.

Box 4.11   Summary of options for treatment of endometriosis

1. No treatment
2. Combined oral contraceptive pill given continuously
3. Oral medroxyprogesterone acetate
4. Danazol
5. GnRH analogues together with 'add back' hormone replacement therapy
6. Laparoscopy and diathermy to endometriosis
7. Laparoscopy and laser ablation of endometriosis
8. Laparotomy/laparoscopy ovarian cystectomy
9. Laparotomy, total abdominal hysterectomy, bilateral salpingo-oophorectomy

It is important to remember that danazol and the combined use of GnRH analogues together with 'add back' hormone replacement therapy are *not* contraceptive measures and the patient should be counselled appropriately. Also oestrogen replacement therapy in a woman who has undergone total abdominal hysterectomy and bilateral salpingo-oophorectomy for pelvic endometriosis may increase the risk of recurrence of endometriosis.

DYSFUNCTIONAL UTERINE BLEEDING

Definition
Dysfunctional uterine bleeding is defined as abnormal bleeding from the uterus in the absence of pregnancy, tumour or inflammation.

Clinical terminology
It is best to describe in plain English exactly what the patient is complaining of or what she is concerned about. The term menorrhagia means heavy periods. The history of heavy cyclical menstrual blood loss over several consecutive cycles should be obtained. Women with intermenstrual bleeding or post-coital bleeding often have underlying organic disease and the symptoms should be described accurately. Metropathia haemorrhagica is usually associated with cystic endometrial hyperplasia and the patient typically complains of a period of amenorrhoea followed by episodes of heavy vaginal bleeding. Polymenorrhoea means that the patient has frequent menstrual periods and oligomenorrhoea means that the patient has infrequent periods.

Clinical investigations
There is some evidence that an abdominal and pelvic examination should be performed in all women complaining of heavy menstrual bleeding. It is also very important to obtain a full blood count in patients complaining of heavy

periods in order to determine whether or not the patient has developed iron deficiency anaemia. Hypothyroidism is associated with menorrhagia and it is important to consider symptoms and signs of the condition. If the patient has clinical features such as hoarseness of the voice, loss of hair, sinus bradycardia and a feeling of being cold then it would be wise to measure the serum TSH (thyroid stimulating hormone).

Referral for further investigations

As a rule it is wise to determine the histological state of the endometrium in any woman who experiences heavy menstrual bleeding at the age of 40 years or above. The reason for this is to determine or exclude the presence of an endometrial tumour. However there are other causes of heavy menstrual bleeding and they include:

- Sub-mucous fibroids
- Intrauterine contraceptive device
- Endometrial polyps
- Adenomyosis
- Chronic pelvic sepsis
- Blood dyscrasias

One of the single most important facts to establish in the management of women with abnormal uterine bleeding is to answer the question – is the uterus normal in size? An enlarged uterus indicates the presence of an organic condition such as a sub-mucous uterine fibroid or adenomyosis, whereas dysfunctional uterine bleeding is associated with a normal-sized uterus. Ultrasound examination of the pelvis is useful as it would assist in answering the following questions of clinical importance.

1. What is the size of the uterus?
2. What is the extent of endometrial thickening?
3. Are there any adnexal masses?
4. Do the ovaries appear to be normal?
5. Does the patient have a hitherto undetected pregnancy?

The woman with irregular vaginal bleeding may well be pregnant and not realize it. As a generalization, the younger the patient the more likely the possibility of a hitherto undetected pregnancy.

Investigating the endometrium

This is a specialist area but it is important that the GP understands the principles so that the patient may be given the proper guidance and explanations.

The following methods are commonly used:

- Examination under anaesthesia (EUA), hysteroscopy and dilatation and curettage (D and C)

- Outpatient diagnostic hysteroscopy and endometrial biopsy
- Ultrasound of the pelvis

EUA, hysteroscopy and D and C remain the gold standard for examining the endometrium. The operation of D and C alone is now outdated: EUA, hysteroscopy and D and C are usually performed on the basis of a day-case unless the patient has underlying anaesthetic or medical complications. The operation takes approximately 10 minutes to perform and complications are usually minimal. Various hospitals in the UK have developed clinics where the patients can undergo outpatient hysteroscopy with endometrial biopsy. Such a procedure is made feasible by the narrow diameter of modern hysteroscopes that enable an excellent view of the uterine cavity with minimal discomfort to the patient. Outpatient endometrial biopsy (without hysteroscopy) using various devices to sample the endometrium is relatively easy to perform and avoids the need for a more formal procedure. However, the presence of a serious lesion may be missed completely in over half the patients.

The following methods of investigating the endometrium are being assessed:

- Three-dimensional ultrasound scanning
- Doppler analysis of blood flow in the pelvis
- Saline infusion sonography

Medical treatment

The following pharmacological agents are useful in the medical treatment of menorrhagia.

- Mefenamic acid
- Tranexamic acid
- Combined oral contraceptive pill
- Depo-medroxyprogesterone acetate

Medical treatment is usually the first line in the treatment of women with dysfunctional uterine bleeding. There may, however, be other relevant factors that influence the decision on management and these include:

- The patient's attitude to her fertility
- History of abnormal cervical smears
- Extent of iron deficiency anaemia (if any)
- Impact of the symptoms on the patient's occupation
- Impact of the symptoms on the patient's lifestyle and social interactions

The following are no longer considered to be effective treatments for menorrhagia: low-dose norethisterone given during the luteal phase, and etamsylate at currently recommended doses.

Progesterone-releasing IUCD

A progesterone releasing intrauterine contraceptive device provides contraception and is an effective treatment for menorrhagia. The Mirena

---

intrauterine system contains 52 mg levonorgestrel and is designed to release 20 μg levonorgestrel within the uterus over a 24-hour period. There is no significant alteration in either the lipid profile or renal function. Reduction of menstrual blood loss following the insertion of a progesterone-releasing IUCD is significant (up to 90%) and may obviate the need for invasive surgery. One of the most important issues to discuss with the patient is the fact that most women experience irregular vaginal bleeding for 8–10 weeks following the insertion of a progesterone-coated IUCD. The Mirena needs to be replaced after five years.

Endometrial ablation
Various innovative techniques have been developed to ablate the endometrium and reduce menstrual blood loss. These procedures need to be performed under general anaesthesia and there is a risk of uterine perforation, haemorrhage and sepsis. The different methods of endometrial ablation include:

- Endometrial resection by loop diathermy
- Rollerball ablation
- Laser ablation
- Microwave ablation
- Balloon ablation
- Cryo ablation

The selection and counselling of patients for such procedures is clearly up to the specialist. The Academy of Medical Royal Colleges has established a safety and efficacy register for new interventional procedures (SERNIP). The SERNIP classification categorizes procedures into four main groups:

1. Safety and efficacy established;
2. Safety and efficacy almost established to the point where there are no reasonable grounds for questioning;
3. Safety and efficacy not yet established;
4. Safety and efficacy shown to be unsatisfactory.

Certain procedures such as endometrial ablation by loop diathermy, rollerball or laser are well established. You may wish to consult the SERNIP classification for other procedures.

It is important to advise patients that endometrial ablation is not a minor operation. In addition to the possible complications listed previously some patients who undergo endometrial ablation by loop diathermy, rollerball or laser may develop fluid overload. The actual procedure is carried out through a fluid medium within the uterus and fluid retention leading to circulatory overload may occur. The success rate of endometrial ablative procedures varies from 65–80%.

Hysterectomy
This type of surgery is best reserved for patients in whom medical treatment has failed. Invariably patients would have undergone an endometrial ablative

procedure but the symptoms either recur or remain. Hysterectomy relieves the patient of the symptoms of dysfunctional uterine bleeding with certainty; it is however a major operation and the risks must be emphasized to the patient (see p. 148 for a full discussion on hysterectomy). It is not necessary to remove the ovaries if hysterectomy is being performed for benign disease of the uterus, although gynaecologists do raise the option of prophylactic bilateral oophorectomy if a hysterectomy is being considered for a woman above the age of 45 years.

UTERINE FIBROIDS

The uterine fibroid is a benign tumour of the smooth muscle of the uterus. It is the most common pelvic tumour and approximately one in four women has a uterine fibroid. There is a tremendous variation in the size of fibroids and in the symptoms that they may produce. Most often the woman is asymptomatic.

Pathology

A uterine fibroid is hormone dependent; it enlarges during pregnancy and regresses following the menopause. Fibroids are often described by their position within the uterus; sub-mucus, intramural or sub-serous. Sub-serous fibroids may become pedunculated and sub-mucus fibroids may be associated with menorrhagia. The following complications may arise:

1. Hyaline degeneration with aseptic necrosis secondary to ischaemia as the fibroid outgrows its blood supply
2. Cystic degeneration preceded by hyaline degeneration
3. Fatty degeneration
4. Red degeneration occurs more frequently in pregnancy or the puerperium
5. Sarcomatous change is extremely rare.

It is important to note that fibroids may arise in the cervix or the ovary. Rarely a fibroid obtains a blood supply from an adjacent organ, loses its blood supply from the uterus and becomes attached to another organ. Such a lesion is termed a 'wandering' fibroid. Although fibroids are benign the extremely rare condition of metastasizing intravenous leiomyomatosis has been described. A fibroid which is pedunculated may undergo torsion.

Clinical features

The patient may well be asymptomatic. However uterine fibroids may be associated with:

- Menorrhagia
- Secondary dysmenorrhoea
- A feeling of abdominal bloatedness

- Pelvic discomfort
- Increased frequency of micturition
- Urinary incontinence secondary to pressure on the bladder (by the enlarged uterus) during coughing or sneezing
- Symptoms of iron deficiency anaemia secondary to menorrhagia

Uterine enlargement secondary to a fibroid may be suspected by the detection of an enlarged uterus on bimanual palpation. Unless the fibroid is huge a fibroid uterus is usually mobile on bimanual palpation. Often the differential diagnosis between a fibroid and adnexal enlargement may be difficult to determine on clinical examination alone.

Investigations
Ultrasound examination of the pelvis is usually able to determine the diagnosis. More sophisticated forms of pelvic imaging include CAT or MRI but such modalities are rarely necessary in the diagnosis of a uterine fibroid.

Management
An asymptomatic woman or a patient with minimal symptoms may be managed conservatively. There is evidence that the use of GnRH analogues may substantially reduce the size of the fibroid and reduce blood loss at a subsequent operation. Indications for surgical intervention include the following:

1. The severity of the patient's symptoms;
2. Iron deficiency anaemia secondary to menorrhagia due to the presence of uterine fibroids;
3. If the uterine size is larger than the clenched fist of an adult;
4. If there is evidence of uterine enlargement over a 3–6 month period.

Surgical intervention may take the form of either abdominal myomectomy or total abdominal hysterectomy, with or without conservation of the ovaries. The choice of operation depends on the discussion between the patient and the specialist she is referred to. However it is important for you as her GP to note that:

- Both abdominal myomectomy and abdominal hysterectomy are major operations with a significant risk of blood loss.
- Abdominal hysterectomy may become necessary during the course of myomectomy in order to control blood loss adequately.
- Abdominal myomectomy may well involve opening the endometrial cavity.
- Abdominal myomectomy ensures preservation of the uterus but the patient would need special care if she were to become pregnant following the operation.
- There is a risk of uterine fibroids following abdominal myomectomy.

Each operation has its advantages and drawbacks. The option to undergo abdominal myomectomy should be discussed with every woman when surgical intervention in the management of uterine fibroids is being considered. Myomectomy should not be performed at the time of Caesarean section as the bleeding may be catastrophic.

GENITOURINARY PROLAPSE

Genitourinary prolapse in women is a common condition. The GP must be able to recognize the clinical symptoms and signs of the condition, determine the presence of risk factors, offer the appropriate non-surgical treatment and refer patients to a specialist as necessary for surgical intervention.

Risk factors
The following conditions predispose to the development of genitourinary prolapse.

- Advancing age
- Post-menopausal change
- Chronic cough
- Constipation
- Occupation involving routine lifting of heavy objects
- Obesity
- Abdominal/pelvic tumour
- Ascites
- Intrinsic weakness of the tissues, for example with Ehlers–Danlos syndrome

Pathology
The supporting tissues of the vagina, cervix, bladder and uterus are weakened by various factors. For example, a patient who smokes cigarettes may develop a chronic cough leading to repeated strain on the supporting ligaments of the genital tract. With advancing age and post-menopausal changes a genitourinary prolapse develops. There are several different types of vaginal prolapse and it is important to realize that two or more types of prolapse may well be present in the same patient. The following is a list of different types of prolapse:

1. Urethrocele
2. Cystocele
3. Rectocele
4. Enterocele
5. Uterine prolapse
6. Vault prolapse (in a patient who has previously undergone hysterectomy).

Clinical symptoms
As a generalization, patients with prolapse of the anterior wall of the vagina tend to develop urinary tract symptoms and those with prolapse of the

posterior wall of the vagina tend to develop symptoms attributable to the gastrointestinal tract. Almost all patients with genitourinary prolapse experience some degree of vaginal or pelvic discomfort and it is important for the general practitioner to be able to elicit this type of symptom from the history. The following is a list of symptoms that a patient with genitourinary prolapse may develop:

1. 'Something coming down'
2. Bulge 'like a ball' at the introitus
3. Increased frequency of micturition
4. Constipation
5. Discomfort during coitus
6. 'Something dangling between the legs'
7. Post-menopausal bleeding from decubitus ulceration of the vagina in patients with complete procidentia.

Clinical signs and classification of prolapse

Following a general and abdominal examination it is important to examine patients in the left lateral position using a Sim's speculum. It is a standard practice to ask the patient to cough while in the left lateral position in order to assess whether or not stress incontinence of urine is present and to assess prolapse of the anterior wall of the vagina. It is also important to ask patients to 'bear down' – as though they were about to open their bowels – in order to assess prolapse of the posterior vaginal wall (rectocele and enterocele). The patient is examined with a Sim's speculum in the left lateral position and asked to bear down while the speculum is slowly removed from the vagina. Some specialists cover the patient's anus while this particular procedure is being carried out so that the patient is able to bear down without inadvertent defaecation. During a specialist examination a volsellum may be used to grip the cervix to gently exert downward traction in order to investigate the degree of uterine prolapse. Such a procedure is uncomfortable for the patient and is best left to a specialist. Descent of the uterus is graded as follows:

Grade 1 – descent of the cervix into the vagina from its usual position
Grade 2 – descent of the cervix to the level of the introitus
Grade 3 – descent of the cervix beyond the introitus
Grade 4 – procidentia. The uterine fundus lies outside the level of the introitus.

A rectal examination may be carried out. The importance of excluding risk factors such as the presence of a pelvic tumour or ascites cannot be over-emphasized. In some patients an ultrasound examination of the abdomen and the pelvis may be very useful.

Treatment

The GP must seek to modify the presence of risk factors such as those listed in the preceding section on risk factors. Patients must be encouraged to lose weight by dieting and to stop smoking cigarettes. The appropriate advice should be given concerning strenuous occupation that involves the lifting of heavy weights. Straining to relieve constipation is a risk factor which can be overcome by dietary modifications, the consumption of adequate amounts of clear fluids and the use of simple laxatives.

There has been a trend to operate on women with genitourinary prolapse rather than use a mechanical pessary in order to control the lesion. There are several reasons for this and they include:

- The risks of surgery and anaesthesia have decreased considerably over the years
- Surgery may produce a 'permanent' cure to the problem
- Many patients would rather undergo surgery when they are relatively young and reasonably fit rather than face the prospect of surgery following the development of cardiopulmonary disease
- There has been a recognition that retained pessaries produce chronic irritation of the vaginal mucosa and in exceptional cases may lead to the development of vaginal carcinoma.

It is important to realize that a vaginal pessary for the control of prolapse should be changed every 3–6 months. A clean pessary should be reinserted after a careful inspection of the vagina to exclude the development of chronic irritation, ulceration and vaginal carcinoma. The patient may be reassured that no special toilet procedures are necessary once a vaginal pessary is inserted for the control of prolapse.

The surgical treatment of patients with genitourinary prolapse is based on the general surgical principle of correcting a hernia anywhere in the body.

1. Resect the redundant epithelium, in this case the vaginal skin
2. Reduce the organ (or part thereof) which has prolapsed
3. Repair the deficiency.

Surgical treatment for genitourinary prolapse is a major undertaking. The GP should refer the patient to the specialist who would then assess the extent of vaginal prolapse and speak to the patient about the appropriate operation (see p. 149 for a list of operations for vaginal prolapse).

Special points for counselling
It is important to note that surgical treatment for vaginal prolapse inevitably leads to narrowing and shortening of the vagina. Colpoperineorrhaphy involves reconstruction of the perennial body and patients commonly report that they can feel 'a muscle' at the fourchette which 'was not there previously'. It is a mistake to assume that elderly patients are not as sexually active and hence the appropriate counselling must be given to any patient who wishes to consider surgery for vaginal prolapse. The appropriate counselling should include the following points:

1. The effect of the operation on the vagina
2. The operation is being performed for vaginal prolapse and not for example for associated symptoms such as urinary incontinence (see below).
3. The duration of inpatient stay
4. The need to avoid or minimize the risk factors post-operatively as well as pre-operatively
5. A vaginal pack may be inserted for 1–2 days post-operatively
6. An indwelling Foley catheter would be inserted toward the end of the operation and left *in situ* for up to 5–6 days post-operatively depending on the actual operation performed and the surgeon's preference
7. There is a risk of urinary tract infection following surgery
8. There is a risk of secondary haemorrhage approximately 1 week following surgery; the condition usually responds to antibiotics.

URINARY INCONTINENCE IN WOMEN

Urinary incontinence is a common symptom in women and the GP should be familiar with its prevalence, risk factors, causes, pathophysiology and the principles of treatment. The symptom is a distressing one and many women find it embarrassing to complain of. It must be noted, however, that urinary incontinence is to be expected in certain circumstances. For example a woman who is 38 weeks pregnant with the presenting part pressing on the bladder may well develop urinary incontinence. Similarly strenuous exercise with a full bladder can lead to involuntary leakage of urine.

Pathophysiology of urinary incontinence

The bladder is a muscular organ which is lined by transitional epithelium and innervated by the autonomic nervous system with both parasympathetic and sympathetic neurones. The parasympathetic neurones travel through the pelvic nerves from the S2, S3 and S4 nerve roots and the nerve terminals themselves release acetylcholine. The acetylcholine acts on the muscarinic receptors at the neuromuscular junctions within the bladder. There are two main sub-types of muscarinic receptor in the human bladder and these are M2 and M3 receptors. M2 receptors act synergistically with the sympathetic neurones to inhibit the detrusor muscle of the bladder when the bladder is being filled. Stimulation of the M3 receptors with acetylcholine leads to contraction of the detrusor muscle at the time of voiding. These mechanisms are subject to control by higher centres through an intact spinal cord.

Urine from the bladder flows out through the urethra which is approximately 4 cm long in women. The urethra is supported by the levator ani muscle and the surrounding ligaments. Urinary continence is maintained by the action of the external urethral sphincter which is subject to voluntary control, the urethral smooth muscle, surrounding collagen and mucosal coarctation of the lining of the urethra.

Women with a weakness of the structures maintaining urinary continence may develop stress incontinence of urine and these risk factors include:

1. High parity
2. Advancing age
3. Menopausal oestrogen deficiency
4. Increased intra-abdominal pressure
5. Trauma to the pelvic floor
6. Connective tissue disease

Cigarette consumption may lead to a chronic cough which gradually damages the supporting structures. Increased abdominal pressure may occur due to coughing, straining during constipation and lifting heavy objects. The presence of a pelvic tumour or ascites may also increase the intra-abdominal pressure to a point where the urethral closing pressure is exceeded and urinary incontinence occurs. Basically the pressure inside the bladder exceeds the pressure in the urethra and urine flows out. A similar situation may occur when the normal voluntary control of the bladder muscle is lost. Under such circumstances the detrusor muscle of the bladder contracts and voluntary inhibition is not achieved. Urinary tract infection is a common underlying factor in incontinent women.

Causes of urinary incontinence
You should be able to recognize urinary incontinence by noting the appropriate symptoms in the history and by examining the patient. For most women referral to a specialist is necessary. Indeed the specialist may have to carry out, arrange or refer to a tertiary centre for urodynamic investigations. These enable a specific and objective diagnosis to be established. The main causes of urinary incontinence are as follows:

1. Urinary fistula
2. Genuine stress incontinence
3. Detrusor instability
4. Mixed – genuine stress incontinence *and* detrusor instability
5. Retention with overflow incontinence
6. Loss of control by higher centres leading to reflex incontinence

The treatment of the condition depends on the diagnosis. The presence of underlying risk factors must be removed or at least modified.

Urinary fistula
A fistula is an abnormal connection between two epithelial surfaces. Various types of urinary fistula may develop and lead to true urinary incontinence. The main causes are:

- Congenital abnormality
- Avascular necrosis secondary to pelvic surgery

- The effects of radiotherapy on the pelvis
- Underlying malignant lesions

Congenital urinary fistulae are extremely rare and should be recognized during the neonatal period, infancy or childhood. Avascular necrosis following pelvic surgery such as abdominal surgery may well lead to a fistula between the urinary tract and the genital tract. Examples of such fistulae include vesicovaginal fistula, uterovaginal fistula, vesicouterine fistula and uretero-uterine fistula.

A urinary fistula must be repaired by a specialist trained to carry out such procedures.

Genuine stress incontinence
Genuine stress incontinence (GSI) is the most common cause of urinary incontinence in women in the UK and the diagnosis is reached in approximately half the women who undergo urodynamic investigations. GSI is defined as the involuntary loss of urine per urethra due to a rise in the intravesical pressure in the absence of detrusor contraction. Approximately 1 in 15 of patients with urinary incontinence will have a mixture of both GSI and detrusor instability. The diagnosis of GSI is established following a urodynamic investigative procedure termed dual-channel subtracted cystometry.

The following non-surgical methods may be used in the initial management of a women with GSI.

- Pelvic floor exercises
- Hormone replacement therapy
- Electrical stimulation
- Biofeedback devices

Pelvic floor exercises, biofeedback and electrical stimulation should be carried out by a suitably trained and qualified physiotherapist. Various 'devices' which have been used to control GSI in women include vaginal cones, pessaries and a urethral cap.

Surgical procedures include anterior colporrhaphy (in the presence of a significant uterovaginal prolapse), abdominal colposuspension, the insertion of tension-free vaginal tape and the periurethral injections of bulk-enhancing agents. Complex procedures such as the insertion of an artificial urethral sphincter and urinary diversion are best performed by sub-specialists in tertiary centres.

Detrusor instability
Detrusor instability (DI) is defined as the involuntary loss of urine per urethra when the bladder is objectively shown to contract when the woman is attempting to inhibit micturition. The contraction may occur spontaneously or on provocation during filling of the bladder in cystometric investigation.

DI is diagnosed in approximately 40% of women undergoing urodynamic investigations; thus it is the second most common cause of urinary incontinence in women but it is important to note that the prevalence may well be increasing as the condition is associated with advanced age.

It is important to reach an accurate diagnosis of DI and certainly if the patient is scheduled to undergo any form of operative procedure for urinary incontinence. The GP should ask the patient questions such as the nature of urinary loss. The most common symptoms of DI are frequency and urgency of micturition, nocturia and nocturnal enuresis of adult onset. It is important to carry out a neurological assessment with particular reference to dermatomes of S2, S3 and S4.

The diagnosis of DI must be confirmed by a specialist or a sub-specialist who can perform dual-channel subtracted cystometry.

There are various methods of treatment for DI and they are as follows: behavioural therapy/bladder drill, anti-cholinergic drugs, anti-muscarinic drugs and tricyclic anti-depressants.

The sub-specialist has other options for offering treatment but procedures such as augmentation cystoplasty are best left to a tertiary centre.

Anti-cholinergic drugs block the action of acetylcholine on the M2 and M3 receptors but they are not very useful as they have very severe systemic side effects. Oxybutynin is an example of an anti-muscarinic drug; although it is useful for the relief of symptoms, it also has an unfavourable profile of side effects, the most consistently troublesome of which is dryness of the mouth. Tolterodine is an anti-muscarinic agent specific for the M3 receptor. It is highly effective in the treatment of DI and causes fewer systemic side effects.

Retention with overflow incontinence
Chronic (as opposed to acute) retention of urine in women leads to the development of an overfilled bladder that leaks spontaneously. Such patients complain of increased frequency of micturition with small amounts of urine, hesitancy and a poor stream of urine. The outflow of the bladder may be obstructed by previous surgery and adhesions. Such patients can be managed by a specialist and may benefit from intermittent self-catheterization of the bladder.

Reflex incontinence
The loss of control by higher centres will lead to a reflex contraction of the bladder muscles as soon as the bladder becomes filled. Referral to a neurologist and sub-specialist is mandatory in the management of such patients.

Management of patients with urinary incontinence
As in so many examples of modern medical care the management of these patients depends on teamwork. The general practitioner, the specialist, the

sub-specialist, the physiotherapist and the continence adviser all have crucial roles to play. The following are indications for urodynamic investigations:

1. The need to establish a diagnosis of GSI, DI or mixed urinary incontinence.
2. All patients scheduled to undergo a surgical procedure for the treatment of GSI.
3. The management of patients who have been treated unsuccessfully (medically or surgically) and who wish to receive further treatment.

The GP should be in a position to take an adequate and relevant history, examine the patient to determine the presence of any prolapse (see p. 135), perform a relevant neurological examination and exclude the presence of urinary tract infection and diabetes mellitus. Following the initial assessment it is best to refer women with urinary incontinence to a specialist.

GYNAECOLOGICAL MALIGNANCY

The general practitioner must recognize the symptoms that may indicate the presence of a gynaecological malignancy, be able to refer patients to a specialist on an urgent basis and be aware of the principles of diagnosis, staging, treatment and prognosis. The GP must also be able to counsel the patient in general terms and support her relatives.

It is useful to remember the following:

1. Post-menopausal bleeding is carcinoma of the endometrium until proved otherwise.
2. Post-coital bleeding is carcinoma of the cervix until proved otherwise.
3. Abdominal distension in a middle-aged or elderly woman is an ovarian tumour until proved otherwise.
4. An ulcer on the vulva of an elderly woman is vulval cancer until proved otherwise.

Histological examination of an adequate biopsy is mandatory before the diagnosis of gynaecological malignancy is established. The lesion must also be staged and most specialists in the UK use the FIGO system of staging.

Carcinoma of the cervix
This lesion is a squamous carcinoma that tends to affect women over the age of 40 years. However it is important to recognize that younger women may also be affected. Risk factors for carcinoma of the cervix include:

- Young age at first coitus
- Multiple sexual partners
- Cigarette consumption
- High parity
- History of sexually transmitted disease including genital wart virus infection.

A patient with squamous carcinoma of the cervix may complain of the following symptoms:

- Post-coital bleeding
- Intermenstrual bleeding
- Post-menopausal bleeding
- Vaginal discharge (which may smell offensive)
- Pelvic pain

If you suspect that a patient has a cervical carcinoma then urgent referral to a specialist is mandatory. The specialist will talk to the patient, examine her and arrange for an appropriate biopsy together with *clinical staging*. Procedures used include examination under anaesthesia, hysteroscopy, diagnostic curettage, biopsy of the cervix, cystoscopy, intravenous urography and computerized axial tomography of the abdomen and pelvis.

The treatment for cervical carcinoma depends on the stage of the disease, the age of the patient, her physical fitness and ability to undergo major surgery and the availability of the appropriate resources. Early cervical carcinoma that is limited to the cervix and upper third of the vagina may be treated with very good results either by radical surgery (Wertheim's hysterectomy – see p. 148) or radiotherapy to the pelvis. More advanced stages of cervical carcinoma require radiotherapy to the pelvis and radical surgery is not indicated. If the patient has a cervical adenocarcinoma then radical surgery is the treatment of choice for early stages of the disease.

The side effects of radiotherapy to the pelvis include:

- Nausea
- Diarrhoea
- Damage to the bowel including ischaemic necrosis of the rectum
- Stenosis of the vagina
- Haematuria
- Urinary fistulae
- Development of pelvic adhesions

Although these symptoms and side effects are rare with modern radiotherapy, it is nevertheless important to remember them; it is also important to remember that gynaecological oncologists may choose to combine surgery with radiotherapy depending on the needs of particular patients.

The results of treatment for squamous carcinoma of the cervix range from a 5-year disease free survival rate of 90–100% for patients with early disease to less than 10% for patients who have involvement of the bladder or rectal mucosa at the time of first presentation.

Carcinoma of the endometrium

Endometrial adenocarcinoma tends to affect post-menopausal women with a peak age of approximately 60 years; it can, however, occur in younger and indeed in older women. It is associated with unopposed oestrogen stimulation, which may arise from the following:

- Unopposed oestrogen replacement therapy in a woman with an intact uterus
- Elevated endogenous oestrogen production in obese women
- Late menopause
- Polycystic ovarian syndrome

There is a significant association with nulliparity. An increased risk of endometrial hyperplasia and progression to endometrial adenocarcinoma has been described in women who take tamoxifen as an adjuvant treatment for breast cancer.

The symptoms of adenocarcinoma of the endometrium include post-menopausal bleeding, menorrhagia, intermenstrual bleeding and irregular menstrual bleeding. The uterus can be bulky on pelvic examination but it may also be normal in size or small. Ultrasound examination demonstrates an increased endometrial thickness. A specialist should arrange for the patient to undergo examination under anaesthesia, hysteroscopy and diagnostic curettage of the endometrium.

The treatment for adenocarcinoma of the endometrium is primarily surgical. Patients are advised to undergo total abdominal hysterectomy and bilateral salpingo-oophorectomy. Following the operation the pathologist should determine the depth of myometrial invasion and the patient would normally be seen by a radiotherapist. Unless the depth of invasion of the myometrium has been minimal patients are usually advised to undergo radiotherapy to the pelvis.

As with all types of malignant lesions the prognosis following treatment for endometrial adenocarcinoma depends on the stage at first presentation. The 5-year survival rates for women with endometrial adenocarcinoma confined to the uterine corpus treated by surgery and radiotherapy are in the order of 90–95%.

Ovarian cancer

Ovarian cancer may occur in any age group but there is a peak in incidence in women who are between 60 and 70 years of age. Certain types of familial ovarian cancer with a genetic basis have been described but most cases are sporadic and the aetiology is unknown. An unfortunate feature of ovarian cancer is that two-thirds of the patients tend to have advanced disease at first presentation; the overall results of treatment therefore do not appear to be as good as the results for cervical cancer or endometrial adenocarcinoma.

A patient with ovarian cancer may have some or all of the following symptoms:

- Abdominal distension
- Abdominal pain

- Dyspepsia
- Unilateral swelling of the leg due to venous obstruction
- Deep-vein thrombosis
- Symptoms of generalized lymphadenopathy

Once you have referred the patient to a specialist the appropriate investigations will be carried out in order to diagnose and stage the lesion. Such investigations will include ultrasound examination of the abdomen and pelvis, CAT of the abdomen and pelvis, MRI of the abdomen and pelvis, measurement of ovarian tumour markers in the serum such as serum Ca 125 and (if necessary) Doppler assessment of the venous system in order to confirm or exclude the presence of a deep-vein thrombosis. Paracentesis may be useful in patients with ascites who are experiencing severe abdominal distension and respiratory difficulties; some of the ascitic fluid may also be sent for cytological examination in the laboratory. It must be stressed however that the diagnosis of ovarian cancer is established when the patient undergoes laparotomy, staging and debulking.

The current approach to the treatment of patients with ovarian cancer is radical surgery followed by cytotoxic chemotherapy. It is important that the primary surgery is undertaken by a gynaecological oncologist or the lead gynaecological cancer surgeon in any particular unit. Patients with ovarian cancer need to undergo *surgical* staging and maximum cyto-reductive surgery – in other words as much tumour as possible should be removed. Patients require omentectomy, and there may be a need for the excision of tumour nodules from various parts of the pelvis and abdomen in addition to total abdominal hysterectomy and bilateral salpingo-oophorectomy. Post-operative cytotoxic chemotherapy for patients with ovarian cancer can include various regimens; considerable experience has been established with the use of platinum-based compounds and the results of treatment with more modern agents such as paclitaxel are very encouraging. Cytotoxic chemotherapy may be used in conjunction with stem-cell transfusion or granulocyte stem-cell stimulation factor. It is essential that cytotoxic chemotherapy is provided in the appropriate units and under the supervision of an appropriately trained oncologist.

Radiotherapy of ovarian tumours may be used in patients who have a 'radio-sensitive' tumour, such as a dysgerminoma.

The overall 5-year survival rate for patients with ovarian cancer is approximately 30%.

Counselling

The general practitioner must play a supportive role in the overall management of patients with gynaecological malignancy. It is important to remember that the patient will go through various phases in receiving bad news: denial, anger, a gradual acceptance and possibly depression. It is essential to allow adequate time for counselling such patients, whether it is

- *Anger.* The patient may well ask the question 'Why me?'. Although they may not ask such a question overtly, many of the reactions, statements and feelings that may be expressed are an indirect expression of this anger.
- *Fear.* The patient may be afraid of various issues including cancer itself, dying, surgery, chemotherapy, radiotherapy and her family's response.
- *Uncertainty.* A patient's self-confidence is shattered following the diagnosis of a malignant lesion. A previously fit person who is told that she has a malignant lesion may find it difficult to accept that anything can be taken as a certainty.
- *Exhaustion.* The lesion itself may cause the patient to feel tired, either by producing anaemia or by reducing her wellbeing – even in the absence of anaemia. It is important to realize that the patient feels exhausted following numerous visits to the hospital, multiple admissions for radiotherapy and/or chemotherapy and following surgery.

to break the initial news of the diagnosis or to answer their subsequent questions. The importance of an adequate amount of time for such patients cannot be over-emphasized. It is also important to speak to the relatives and play a supportive role in helping them through a very difficult period. Patients with gynaecological malignancy develop a variety of reactions and Box 4.12 describes some of them.

Terminal care

The multi-disciplinary team that manages the patient with gynaecological malignancy must make the difficult decision as to whether or not the patient has a terminal illness as a result of this. The patient herself may – after consultation with her family – request that treatment is avoided. Depending on the conditions that are present and the availability of resources the patient may elect to stay at home, be admitted to a local hospice or admitted to a hospital ward. It is important to provide the patient with adequate pain relief, expert nursing support and adequate nutrition as a part of terminal care.

GYNAECOLOGICAL OPERATIONS

A GP is not required to perform gynaecological operations but as a GP, you would be expected to be able to counsel patients regarding some of the more general issues concerning such operations. The following is a description of operations commonly performed by gynaecologists together with explanatory notes and information that patients will find useful.

Examination under anaesthesia, hysteroscopy and diagnostic curettage
Although there is a move to perform diagnostic hysteroscopy on an outpatient basis under local anaesthesia the operation of examination under anaesthesia (EUA), hysteroscopy and diagnostic curettage (dilatation and curettage – D and C) is one of the more commonly performed gynaecological operations. The purpose of the EUA is to assess the vulva, vagina, cervix, the size, position and mobility of the uterus, the adnexa, the Pouch of Douglas, the contents of the rectum and the degree of descent of the cervix and the uterus with gentle downward traction. The purpose of performing a hysteroscopy is to directly visualize the endometrial cavity with particular reference to the endometrium itself. The gynaecologist would identify the cornual orifices and systematically examine the fundus and anterior, posterior and lateral walls of the uterine cavity. Hysteroscopy may be performed either through a fluid or a gaseous medium. The diagnostic curettage is performed in order to obtain material for endometrial biopsy and to remove any polyps which may be present.

Unless the patient is beyond a certain age or she has problems which may increase the risk of complications of anaesthesia the operation of EUA, hysteroscopy and D and C is commonly performed as a day-case procedure. The patient should be given a simple description of the operation, its purpose and potential complications which include bleeding, infection and uterine perforation. If the operation is being carried out as a day-case procedure the patient should be accompanied home by a member of the family or a close friend. A small amount of vaginal bleeding, which may last for 5–6 days post-operatively, is expected in most cases.

Large loop excision of the transformation zone (LLETZ)
This particular procedure is a means of obtaining a loop excision biopsy of the cervix (see p. 119). The procedure is most commonly performed under local anaesthesia and on an outpatient basis. However, some patients may prefer to undergo the procedure under general anaesthesia. The lesion may be vascular, hence increasing the risk of post-procedural blood loss, or it may be very extensive: under such circumstances the LLETZ operation should be performed under general anaesthesia.

Cone biopsy of the cervix
Diagnostic conization of the cervix using the scalpel (as opposed to laser or the loop diathermy) is performed under general anaesthesia and classified as an 'intermediate' operation. Cone biopsy of the cervix is *not* a minor procedure. The indications for cone biopsy of the cervix include: inconclusive colposcopy, unsatisfactory colposcopy (where the squamo-columnar junction cannot be visualized adequately), discrepancy between histological and colposcopic findings, a lesion that extends into the endocervical canal and whose upper limit cannot be seen by colposcopic examination and suspected adenocarcinoma *in situ* within the endocervical

canal. The potential complications of cone biopsy of the cervix include haemorrhage (which may be severe) and sepsis. In a woman of childbearing age complications include cervical incompetence during a subsequent pregnancy or cervical stenosis leading to cervical dystocia (slow progress in cervical dilatation) in labour. Cervical stenosis may also lead to secondary dysmenorrhoea.

Laparoscopy

Gynaecological laparoscopy involves the placement (under general anaesthesia or spinal block) of a needle into the peritoneal cavity, creation of a pneumoperitoneum, insertion of a trochar and finally a laparoscope in order to inspect the pelvis. In diagnostic laparoscopy a second portal of entry is often required so that an appropriate instrument may be used to manipulate the uterus while the operator inspects the area through the laparoscope. In operative laparoscopy a total of three or possibly four portals of entry may be required in order to insert various instruments including diathermy electrodes, laparoscopic scissors, sutures and manipulating instruments.

There are various indications for diagnostic laparoscopy including the investigation of pelvic pain, the need to establish a diagnosis of endometriosis, the need to determine the presence of or exclude a tubal pregnancy, to inspect the uterus and adnexae and to investigate infertility. The operation of 'laparoscopy and dye' test includes the insertion of a transcervical cannula into the uterine cavity and the injection of sterile methylene-blue dye into the uterus. Bilateral tubal patency or indeed tubal occlusive disease may be easily diagnosed. Laparoscopic sterilization includes the operation of diagnostic laparoscopy, appropriate manipulation of the uterus and the insertion of an occlusive device to each of the Fallopian tubes (see p.175). Appropriately selected patients may undergo diagnostic laparoscopy, laparoscopy and dye test and operations for laparoscopic sterilization as a day-case procedure. It is important to remember that obesity is both a surgical and anaesthetic hazard and patients with a body mass index above a certain limit may not necessarily be able to undergo day-case surgery. Patients who undergo laparoscopy should be given the following information:

- A simple description of the procedure
- The purpose of the procedure
- The risk of injury to the urinary tract
- The risk of injury to the bowel – approximately 1 in 1000
- The risk of bleeding
- The risk of infection
- The need for a suitable anaesthetic.

It is also important to remember that patients may develop emotional responses following invasive procedures such as laparoscopy.

Abdominal hysterectomy

Abdominal hysterectomy is one of the most commonly performed elective operations in the UK. The operation involves removal of the body of the uterus and the cervix. Sub-total hysterectomy involves removal of the body of the uterus and conservation of the cervix. Either operation may be combined with bilateral salpingo-oophorectomy – removal of the Fallopian tubes and ovaries. Wertheim's hysterectomy involves removal of the uterus, cervix (+/- salpingo-oophorectomy) and pelvic lymphadenectomy involving dissection of the ureteric tunnel and exploration of the iliac and obturator lymph nodes.

In addition to the operative hazards and the risks of general anaesthesia it is important to realize that patients who undergo abdominal hysterectomy are at a significant risk of developing post-operative deep-vein thrombosis (DVT) and pulmonary embolism. Various prophylactic measures should be taken by the specialist and the team who are managing the patient in the secondary or tertiary care centre, but it is important for the GP to recognize the significance of any symptom of dyspnoea or chest pain in a patient who has recently undergone pelvic surgery.

The GP should be able to convey the information in Box 4.13 to patients who are scheduled to undergo abdominal hysterectomy.

As a GP you will not be directly involved in issues such as the choice of abdominal incision. Any of the aforementioned operations for hysterectomy may be performed, either through a transverse lower abdominal incision, a midline incision or a paramedian incision of the abdomen.

Vaginal hysterectomy

This operation involves removal of the uterus and cervix through vaginal incisions. It is possible to perform bilateral salpingo-oophorectomy at the time of vaginal hysterectomy although most specialists leave the ovaries *in*

Box 4.13   Information needed by abdominal hysterectomy patients

- A simple description of the procedure
- The purpose of the operation
- The need for appropriate anaesthesia
- The risk of haemorrhage
- The risk of infection
- The risk of injury to the urinary tract
- The risk of injury to the gastrointestinal tract
- The risk of post-operative DVT and pulmonary embolism
- It can take up to 4–6 weeks before the patient can drive a car
- The pathology report on the operation specimen should be discussed with the patient in due course
- It will take 2–3 months for the patient to resume an active lifestyle

---

situ provided the organs look and feel normal at the time of the vaginal hysterectomy.

Complications of vaginal hysterectomy are similar to those listed under 'Abdominal hysterectomy' in the preceding section. On the whole patients tend to recover more speedily following vaginal hysterectomy than abdominal hysterectomy.

Anterior colporrhaphy

This is an operation performed for the surgical correction of a cystocele. The redundant vaginal skin in the anterior vaginal wall is excised, the bladder is returned to its normal position and the paravesical and paraurethral tissues are sutured in place in order to prevent a recurrence of the cystocele. Postoperative Foley catheterization of the bladder is commonly required for a few days.

Colpoperineorrhaphy

This is an operation for surgical correction of a rectocele. The redundant vaginal skin is excised, the rectum is replaced into its normal position and the levator ani muscles are sutured so as to prevent a recurrence of the rectocele.

The operation of colpoperineorrhaphy may be combined with anterior colporrhaphy or vaginal hysterectomy depending on the degree and nature of prolapse (see p. 134).

Laparoscopically assisted vaginal hysterectomy

In this procedure operative laparoscopy is combined with a vaginal hysterectomy in order to remove the uterus and cervix (+/- Fallopian tubes and ovaries) vaginally. The time taken for recovery following laparoscopically assisted vaginal hysterectomy is significantly shorter than standard abdominal hysterectomy. This particular operation is only performed by certain specialists in certain centres.

Choice of route for hysterectomy

There are various reasons why a specialist and patient may decide on a certain route for hysterectomy and these may be summarized as follows: necessity, feasibility and preference.

If the patient has a large ovarian tumour it would be wise to perform laparotomy through a long midline abdominal incision. On the other hand if the patient has a procidentia (see p. 135) it would be a relatively easy procedure for an appropriately trained specialist to perform the operation of vaginal hysterectomy and either anterior colporrhaphy or colpoperineorrhaphy. Some surgeons prefer a certain route such as a laparoscopically assisted vaginal hysterectomy or standard vaginal as opposed to abdominal hysterectomy and the appropriate issues should be discussed with individual patients.

Myomectomy

This operation involves resection of a fibroid from the uterus. There is a significant risk of bleeding and specialists commonly counsel the patient concerning the need to perform abdominal hysterectomy if the bleeding from the site of the excised fibroid cannot be controlled.

Ovarian cystectomy

This is an operation that is performed for benign cysts of the ovary. The benign cyst is removed and sent for histological examination. Depending on its size, position and level of adherence to the surrounding structures the operation may be performed either by open laparotomy or laparoscopically.

Salpingectomy, salpingostomy and salpingotomy

Salpingectomy is the surgical resection of the Fallopian tube. The term salpingostomy applies to the operation for unblocking the fimbrial end of the Fallopian tube, while salpingotomy refers to the operation whereby the Fallopian tube is incised and left open; the operation is one of the procedures which may be performed as a treatment for a tubal ectopic pregnancy when it would be beneficial to conserve the affected Fallopian tube. Operations on the Fallopian tube may be performed either laparoscopically or by open laparotomy.

COMPLICATIONS IN EARLY PREGNANCY

There are four complications in early pregnancy of which the general practitioner must be aware and these are: abortion, ectopic pregnancy, molar pregnancy and bleeding from lesions in the lower genital tract. Although vaginal bleeding is a hallmark of complications in early pregnancy the symptom may not necessarily be present: for example, it is possible for a patient to develop a ruptured ectopic pregnancy with massive intraperitoneal haemorrhage without any external bleeding from the vagina. Patients with delayed miscarriage may not have any vaginal bleeding at all, and the diagnosis is not apparent until an ultrasound examination is performed.

Abortion

Abortion is defined as the expulsion of the products of conception before the 24th week of pregnancy. In practice it is considered to be the expulsion of the products of conception before the threshold of fetal viability; this is of course a controversial area as a fetus may survive following expulsion from the uterus as early as 20 or 21 weeks.

Spontaneous miscarriage includes the following:

- Threatened miscarriage
- Delayed miscarriage (missed abortion)
- Inevitable miscarriage which may be complete or incomplete

Causes of spontaneous miscarriage

1. Fetal abnormalities: chromosomal abnormalities, congenital malformations and abnormalities of the fetal membranes
2. Cervical incompetence
3. Congenital malformation of the uterus
4. Pelvic tumours such as uterine fibroids
5. Trauma to the uterus
6. Maternal illness, especially in the presence of fever, untreated syphilis, severe hypertension and chronic renal disease
7. Drug ingestion: ergot and quinine

Prevalence

Spontaneous miscarriage is common. During the latter part of the first trimester approximately 20% of all pregnancies result in a spontaneous miscarriage. The prevalence is even higher in earlier stages of gestation.

Clinical features

The main symptom of threatened miscarriage is vaginal bleeding. The patient usually reports a period of amenorrhoea prior to the vaginal bleeding. Other symptoms of early pregnancy such as nausea and vomiting, breast tenderness and increased frequency of micturition may also be present in the history. The patient may also complain of uterine contractions. It is important to note that the amount of vaginal bleeding in patients with spontaneous miscarriage may be considerable.

On clinical examination you should note the presence of blood in the vagina; the cervical os would be closed in cases of threatened miscarriage and dilated, possibly with the passage of products of conception, in cases of inevitable miscarriage.

Investigation

The development and application of ultrasound scanning has radically altered the management of patients with bleeding in early pregnancy. Most secondary and tertiary care units have developed early pregnancy assessment units that are staffed by nurses, bereavement support counsellors and ultrasonographers. It is important to note that the investigation of complications of early pregnancy requires adequately trained staff and the appropriate equipment.

An adequate ultrasound examination provides information on the size, shape and regularity of the gestational sac, their number, the presence of one or more fetal poles, whether or not fetal heart pulsations are observed and the presence of an intrauterine haematoma. In patients with equivocal findings it may be necessary to repeat the ultrasound examination 7–10 days later in order to determine whether or not the patient has an ongoing pregnancy.

The measurement of serum beta HCG indicates whether or not the patient has trophoblastic tissue which is producing that particular sub-unit of human chorionic gonadotrophin. Repeated measurements of serum beta HCG may be necessary in order to distinguish between an ongoing intrauterine pregnancy, ectopic pregnancy, delayed miscarriage, complete miscarriage or molar pregnancy. Rather than try and remember prescriptive rules you would be able to interpret the significance of the various findings by remembering the following information:

- Serum beta HCG rises during pregnancy
- There is a wide range in serum beta
- The half-life of HCG in human serum is approximately 48 hours. In other words, if the patient has expelled the trophoblastic tissue in her body or any residual trophoblastic tissue has ceased to function the serum beta HCG would have fallen to half of its value 2 days later.

Management

If a patient has suffered a delayed or incomplete miscarriage, evacuation of retained products of conception under general anaesthesia is offered. It is also important to provide Rhesus negative women with an intramuscular injection of anti-D immunoglobulin 250 IU as soon as possible after the diagnosis has been established. Psychological and emotional support of the patient is extremely important, and many units employ bereavement support counsellors.

It is important to realize that the patient suffers a very real bereavement if she miscarries in early pregnancy, and it is important to acknowledge her sense of loss. The services for investigation and management may well be provided on a fast-track basis with specialized early pregnancy assessment units but the intention is to provide rapid services and not to fast-track the patient. Although the diagnosis may be made promptly it is important to offer the patient a choice of whether or not to undergo surgery the same day or within the next 1–2 days. If the patient passes an identifiable fetus per vaginum it is best to ask her whether or not the fetus may be subjected to a histological examination – even during the first trimester. Many families may wish to arrange a private burial or cremation for the first-trimester fetus.

Septic abortion

A septic abortion results from microbial infection of the genital tract secondary to a spontaneous or induced abortion. It is essential to refer such cases to a specialist. In addition to the clinical features of bleeding in early pregnancy the patient usually develops a fever, offensive-smelling vaginal discharge and pelvic tenderness. Management includes the use of parenteral broad-spectrum antibiotics to cover Gram-negative organisms, intravenous fluids and surgical evacuation of the uterus.

Recurrent abortion

A patient who suffers three spontaneous miscarriages consecutively is said to have a history of recurrent or habitual abortion. The causes of recurrent abortion include:

1. Parental chromosomal abnormality in 3–5% of couples with recurrent miscarriage
2. Thrombophilic defects
3. Polycystic ovaries.

Current studies are trying to establish the relationship between bacterial vaginosis and a history of recurrent abortion.

Molar pregnancy

A complete mole is a pregnancy in which there is no fetus and the placental villi undergo hydropic degeneration. A partial mole is a pregnancy in which there is a fetus and molar changes in the placenta.

Incidence   In the UK the incidence of complete moles is 1/1200 deliveries. The true incidence of partial moles is uncertain but most estimates place the order at approximately 1/600 deliveries.

Pathology   Complete moles are diploid with two paternal haplotypes. Partial moles are triploid with three sets of chromosomes: two paternal haplotypes and one maternal haplotype. The term 'hydatidiform' refers to the vesicular changes which occur in the placenta. Hydatidiform moles are composed of vesicular masses and variable degrees of trophoblastic proliferation.

It is extremely important to note that both complete and partial moles may give rise to choriocarcinoma. The incidence of choriocarcinoma following a complete molar pregnancy is approximately 3%. The term 'gestational trophoblastic disease' is applied to the clinical situation when a patient has suffered a hydatidiform mole and has persistent evidence of trophoblastic disease as indicated by elevated serum HCG.

Biochemistry   The main biochemical hallmark of hydatidiform pregnancy is the increased production of HCG. The patient's serum HCG is grossly elevated and continues to rise unless the molar tissue is removed from the patient's body.

Clinical features   The most common presentation of a patient with a molar pregnancy is vaginal bleeding during the second half of the first trimester of pregnancy. Ultrasound examination of the pelvis usually reveals the diagnosis. The serum HCG is significantly elevated. In some cases the serum beta HCG is so high that the HCG molecules adhere to each other and fail to react in the laboratory test; this is termed the 'Hook effect'. If you suspect that a patient has a molar pregnancy it is useful to inform the biochemical laboratory who would then dilute the patient's serum in order to assess the serum beta HCG accurately.

Treatment   Any patient who has a hydatidiform pregnancy must be referred to a secondary or tertiary care centre. The initial treatment is to evacuate the uterus and in some cases a second evacuation may be necessary. It is mandatory to register patients with complete or partial mole onto the national scheme for monitoring beta HCG. There are three reference laboratories that carry out serial measurements of serum HCG at a national level and these are based in Dundee, Sheffield and at the Charing Cross Hospital in London.

In the majority of patients the serum HCG returns to normal; once it has there is no contraindication to the use of the oral contraceptive pill. It has been shown, however, that the use of exogenous hormones, including the oral contraceptive pill, may stimulate the growth of rests of molar tissue.

If the patient develops gestational trophoblastic disease or choriocarcinoma and her serum HCG levels continue to rise the tertiary care centre should manage the patient appropriately. A risk score is performed and the patient is offered either single agent or multiple agent chemotherapy.

Local causes

Bleeding in early pregnancy may occur due to lesions in the lower genital tract such as vulval and vaginal warts, ulcers and lacerations.

ECTOPIC PREGNANCY

Ectopic pregnancy occurs when a fertilized egg implants at a site other than the uterine cavity. The most common site for an ectopic pregnancy is the ampullary portion of a Fallopian tube. Other sites include the cervix, cornual portion of the body of the uterus, ovaries or the pelvic peritoneum.

Significance

The incidence of ectopic pregnancy in the UK is approximately 1 in 80. It is important to note the significance of ectopic pregnancy: it is an important cause of maternal death, and the diagnosis may be particularly difficult to establish.

Aetiology

In many cases the exact cause of the ectopic pregnancy is unknown. Underlying and associated factors include the following:

- A history of tubal surgery
- Pelvic adhesions, secondary to previous surgery, appendicectomy or pelvic inflammatory disease
- Pelvic endometriosis
- Assisted conception
- Pelvic tuberculosis in certain parts of the world

- Previous ectopic pregnancy
- Use of an intrauterine contraceptive device or the progesterone-only pill (debatable).

Clinical features

Approximately 25% of ectopic pregnancies present with the patient in shock. The ectopic pregnancy ruptures and a large haemoperitoneum is created. The patient develops circulatory shock very quickly and the characteristic clinical picture often seen in Accident and Emergency departments includes:

- Evidence of circulatory shock
- Abdominal distension
- Tenderness on abdominal palpation and on pelvic examination
- Low serum Hb

In cases where the presentation is less acute the patient usually complains of the classic 'triad' of symptoms: amenorrhoea, lower abdominal pain and vaginal bleeding.

The patient develops amenorrhoea as the ectopic pregnancy produces human chorionic gonadotrophin which stimulates the ovaries to produce oestrogen and progesterone continuously. As the ectopic pregnancy grows within the Fallopian tube the patient develops abdominal pain secondary to distension of a viscus. Vaginal bleeding occurs when the hormonal support for the endometrium is withdrawn as production of beta HCG by the ectopic pregnancy falters.

The patient may well develop a collection of blood within the pelvis. As the blood accumulates in the Pouch of Douglas, gastrointestinal symptoms such as tenesmus and diarrhoea may develop.

Owing to the chronic accumulation of blood within the pelvis over several days in an undiagnosed and untreated ectopic pregnancy the patient gradually becomes anaemic and experiences attacks of fainting and dizziness.

As the blood from the pelvis tracts up the abdominal cavity and irritates the diaphragm the patient may develop shoulder-tip (referred) pain.

Some patients develop what is called a tubal abortion. In such cases the ectopic pregnancy is expelled from the Fallopian tube and enters the Pouch of Douglas. It is slowly reasorbed and after the initial attack of lower abdominal pain her symptoms gradually resolve. On pelvic examination the patient characteristically exhibits the important clinical sign of localized pelvic tenderness on bimanual examination. On bimanual palpation, if you gently grasp the cervix and move it from side to side the patient complains of tenderness – this is called cervical excitation.

Differential diagnosis

The following conditions may well be confused with an ectopic pregnancy in the Fallopian tubes:

- Appendicitis
- Salpingo-oophoritis

- Acute pyelonephritis
- Ovarian cyst
- Other causes of bleeding in early pregnancy

Investigation
The development and application of ultrasound examination of the pelvis has greatly enhanced our capability for diagnosing ectopic pregnancy. As a useful rule of thumb the combination of a positive pregnancy test or elevated serum beta HCG accompanied by an 'empty' uterus on ultrasound examination is an ectopic pregnancy until proved otherwise. This point cannot be over-emphasized. Diagnostic pitfalls may however arise and the following conditions can produce the same clinical picture: recent complete abortion, or very early intrauterine pregnancy.

The presence of an elevated serum beta HCG in a woman's serum indicates the presence of trophoblastic tissue. In the investigation and management of women suspected of having an unruptured ectopic pregnancy serial measurement of serum beta HCG is often useful in conjunction with ultrasound examination of the pelvis. Serum beta HCG is, however, subject to wide natural variation and undue reliance on a laboratory investigation may lead to problems.

The following will help you to interpret the significance of serum beta HCG: (a) The half-life of serum beta HCG is approximately 48 hours, that is, you would expect the serum beta HCG to halve in 48 hours once trophoblastic tissue is removed from the body; and, (b) the serum level of beta HCG starts to rise at a very early stage in pregnancy and Table 4.1 gives you some idea of the range that may be expected at different stages in gestation.

Table 4.1 Expected range at gestation stages in ectopic pregnancy

Gestation in weeks	Mean serum beta HCG (mIU/ml)	Range (mIU/ml)
3 weeks	25	0.0–100
4 weeks	282	60–1000
5 weeks	26 500	3800–92 000
6 weeks	39 500	3200–96 000
7 weeks	59 000	7000–147 000
8 weeks	98 500	13 750–168 000

Treatment
A patient with a ruptured ectopic pregnancy needs to undergo emergency laparotomy; adequate amounts of blood for transfusion must be available.

A patient with an unruptured ectopic pregnancy should undergo confirmation of the diagnosis by diagnostic laparoscopy; the appropriate operation can then be carried out.

Surgery for ectopic pregnancy has developed from removal of the affected Fallopian tube and ipsilateral ovary to salpingectomy alone, and then to partial salpingectomy. The current approach is to perform laparoscopic treatment for unruptured ectopic pregnancy.

Laparoscopic management of unruptured ectopic pregnancy includes various measures such as laparoscopic salpingectomy, laparoscopic salpingostomy or laparoscopic injection of methotrexate into the ectopic pregnancy.

The treatment of ectopic pregnancy is clearly a highly specialized procedure and one of the most important points to grasp in general practice is to refer the patient for specialist care as soon as an ectopic pregnancy is suspected.

A Rhesus negative woman who has suffered an ectopic pregnancy requires an intramuscular injection of anti-D immunoglobulin.

Counselling

A woman who has suffered an ectopic pregnancy has a higher risk that her subsequent pregnancy will also be complicated by ectopic implantation. Patients need a high level of support and explanation by the hospital staff and primary care team following the emotional and physical stresses associated with management of ectopic pregnancy. This distress includes the following:

- Initial symptoms of pain
- Possible uncertainty of diagnosis
- Disappointment that a planned pregnancy has become very complicated
- Emergency surgery
- Possible need for blood transfusion
- Awareness that an ectopic pregnancy may well occur again in the future

It is crucial to advise all patients with ectopic pregnancy that in the future they should inform their doctor as soon as they know they are pregnant again so that the appropriate investigations to exclude or confirm the diagnosis of an ectopic pregnancy may be carried out.

Many units in the UK have established early pregnancy assessment units in order to assist in the early diagnosis and management of women who are suspected of having an ectopic pregnancy.

TERMINATION OF PREGNANCY

Termination of pregnancy is one of the commonest gynaecological procedures. Around 154 000 terminations are performed annually in England and Wales and around 11 000 in Scotland.

About 99% of terminations are undertaken by NHS staff in Scotland. In England and Wales this proportion is about 55% with a further 16% funded by the NHS through contracts with non-NHS providers.

Remember that the Abortion Act 1967 does not apply to Northern Ireland and about 1500 women annually make the journey to Britain for a termination to be performed. This is usually performed outside the NHS. When performed early in pregnancy, abortion is associated with a lower risk of complications. Early referral is required by law. When suitable, termination should be performed as a day-case service.

Women requesting termination early in pregnancy, at about 9 weeks or less, should be given the choice of either medical or surgical termination.

Antibiotic prophylactic is needed for minimizing the risk of post-abortion infective morbidity.

Determination of blood group and Rhesus factor are essential; anti-D should be given to Rhesus negative women. If clinically indicated, haemoglobin level should be checked post-abortion.

At the time of referral for such a service, enquire about cervical screening and discuss and stress the importance of contraception.

The abortion notification form and maternal consent must be obtained before any termination is attempted.

Surgical termination should be avoided at gestation of ≤6 weeks. At a gestation of 7 weeks or less, medical termination using mifepristone and prostaglandin is the preferred method. Cervical preparation is beneficial prior to suction termination. This should be routine in all girls at 18 years or below and when the gestation is more than 10 weeks.

If she wishes to opt for surgical termination, the woman should be given the choice of local anaesthetic. In the second trimester, medical termination with mifepristone followed by prostaglandin is safe and effective.

Counselling is an essential part of the service of termination. Time should be allowed for discussion and explanation. It is not an easy decision to opt for a termination.

Perforation, bleeding, retained products and infection may complicate surgical termination. Follow-up is required for cases of termination and the general practitioner plays an essential role.

MEDICAL MANAGEMENT OF THE MENOPAUSE

Physiology and biochemistry

The age at which a woman has her final menstrual period is termed the menopause. The period of time around the menopause is termed the climacteric, just as the age at which a woman has her first menstrual period is termed the menarche and the period of time around the menarche is termed puberty. The average age of menopause in the UK is 52 years.

For various demographic reasons the number of post-menopausal women as a proportion of the population is *increasing*.

Oogenesis ceases in the female at 20 weeks in utero. By the time a female is born the number of eggs in the body has dropped from a peak of 7 million to approximately 1 million. By the time the menopause occurs the last egg has been released from the ovary. Following the menopause the serum FSH and LH levels rise significantly as the negative feedback of oestrogen levels on the pituitary is diminished. Serum FSH and LH rise beyond 25 IU/l following the menopause and the serum FSH is usually much higher than the serum LH. The normal range of serum estradiol varies from 50 to 1000 pmol/l and for this reason among others measurement of serum estradiol may be difficult to interpret.

Following the menopause the rate of bone resorption from the skeleton increases. A woman loses approximately 1% of her skeletal bone mass per annum following the menopause. Post-menopausal changes in serum lipids include a rise in low-density lipoprotein cholesterol and a fall in high-density lipoprotein cholesterol.

An oestrogen has traditionally been defined as any substance that increases the weight of the mammalian uterus and causes proliferative changes in the endometrium. Progesterone has traditionally been defined as any substance inducing secretory change in a proliferative endometrium. The current definition of an oestrogen is a substance that binds specifically to an oestrogen receptor, while a progesterone is a substance that binds specifically to a progesterone receptor. More recently different types of oestrogen receptors have been defined and they have varying distributions within the female body. Some types of oestrogen are capable of altering the molecular structure of the oestrogen receptors to which they bind. These substances are called steroid (o)estrogen receptor modulators (SERMs)

It is important to realize that oestrogens, progesterones and SERMs have effects in many different and varied organs and not just in the genital tract.

Management

The concept of hormone replacement therapy (HRT) arose more than 40 years ago. It is intended to replace the amount of oestrogen lost in the body of a post-menopausal woman. The provision of HRT to post-menopausal women has been ranked near the discovery of penicillin in terms of significant medical advances during the twentieth century.

Oestrogen prevents post-menopausal osteoporosis. The use of oral oestrogens in a post-menopausal woman increases serum high-density lipoprotein cholesterol and decreases serum low-density lipoprotein cholesterol. There is also an increase in serum triglycerides. The use of tibolone leads to a marked reduction in serum lipoprotein A and the effect is observed to a lesser extent following treatment with either oral oestrogen or raloxifene (a SERM). The use of transdermal oestrogen replacement therapy leads to a reduction of serum low-density lipoprotein cholesterol and serum triglyceride levels.

Oestrogen causes proliferative changes in the endometrium and if it is used without progesterone in a woman with an intact uterus it increases the risk of endometrial cancer. Therefore if you prescribe oestrogen to a woman

Box 4.14 Benefits of hormone replacement therapy

- Prevention of post-menopausal osteoporosis
- Reduction in the risk of mortality from ischaemic heart disease by approximately 50%
- Relief of climacteric symptoms.

There is some evidence that the following benefits may also be obtained:

- Reduction in the age of onset of Alzheimer's disease
- Reduction in the risk of colorectal cancer.

Absolute contraindications to hormone replacement therapy include the following:

- Irregular and unexplained vaginal bleeding
- Pregnancy
- Significant disease of the liver.

Side effects of oestrogen replacement therapy include vaginal bleeding, breast tenderness and a subjective sense of weight gain. Potential long-term complications include the following:

- Slight increase in the risk of breast cancer following long-term use (more than 5–10 years)
- Slightly increased risk of deep-vein thrombosis and pulmonary embolism.

When you take a history from a woman who is considering hormone replacement therapy it is advisable to ask the following questions:

1. Is there a family history of malignant disease, especially breast cancer?
2. Is there a family history of osteoporosis?
3. Is there a possibility of pregnancy?
4. Is there a history of liver disease?
5. Is there a history of unexplained irregular vaginal bleeding?

with an intact uterus you must also prescribe progesterone. The benefits of hormone replacement therapy are listed in Box 4.14.

The importance of counselling a woman regarding HRT cannot be over-emphasized. You need to take note of the patient's concerns and answer her questions as fully as possible.

The consultation prior to starting HRT provides an important opportunity to perform screening and the measures which you should consider include ensuring that the patient is up to date with her cervical smears, measurement of serum thyroid stimulating hormone (TSH) level and ensuring that the patient has taken up invitations for mammography.

Types of hormone replacement therapy

Oestrogen and progesterone may be prescribed for use in oral tablet form or to be applied as a patch over the skin over the abdomen or the lateral aspect of the thighs.

Combined (oestrogen and progesterone) HRT may be offered in sequential form using either oral tablets or transdermal patches for women with an intact uterus. If a woman has already undergone hysterectomy she may receive either oral or transdermal oestrogen without progesterone. If the woman has been amenorrhoeic for more than 12 months after the menopause and she has an intact uterus a further option would be the use of continuous combined hormone replacement therapy which may be given either as oral tablets or transdermal patches. A further alternative would be the use of tibolone tablets which have oestrogenic, progestogenic and mild androgenic activity.

Oestrogen may also be provided as an implant. However this form of oestrogen replacement therapy leads to a very high serum level of estradiol and is best reserved for women who have developed positive tachyphylaxis to oral or transdermal oestrogen.

Testosterone implants have been used to restore libido in women for whom treatment with oestrogen and progesterone has failed. However this form of treatment requires detailed counselling and is best left to a specialist clinic.

Raloxifene

Raloxifene is a steroid (o)estrogen receptor modulator (SERM). It binds to an oestrogen receptor and alters the molecular structure of the receptor. Raloxifene prevents vertebral stress fractures in women at risk of osteoporosis. It also lowers serum low-density lipoprotein cholesterol and serum lipoprotein A. These biochemical actions are desirable *vis-à-vis* the prevention of ischaemic heart disease. Raloxifene does not prevent climacteric symptoms or reverse atrophy of the vagina in post-menopausal women. The use of raloxifene is contraindicated in women with a history of breast cancer and a history of DVT. It is taken as an oral tablet; the main side effects include nausea and leg cramps.

Points to consider when prescribing HRT

It is important to set common goals with your patient before you prescribe hormone replacement therapy.

In addition to educating your patient you should provide advice on important issues such as the need for regular exercise, dietary advice and the need to stop smoking cigarettes and consuming excessive amounts of alcohol. A woman should be advised to perform weight-bearing exercises (including aerobics and the use of weights) for at least 30 minutes three times a week. Dietary advice should be aimed at reducing the amount of cholesterol consumed and increasing the amount of desirable foods such as white fish, soya products and foods rich in isoflavones and lignans. The patient must be given some simple advice on relaxation techniques and the need to create some time for herself, at least once during each day.

Approximately 5% of women who take oestrogen replacement therapy develop positive tachyphylaxis – an increasing dosage of the same drug is used to create the same therapeutic response. In the case of oestrogen replacement therapy you may find that an increasing dosage of oestrogen is required to control the patient's climacteric symptoms. Such women may well benefit from the use of an implant of oestrogen, initially provided at a dosage of 50 mg estradiol every 6 months.

Post-menopausal hormone replacement therapy should be continued on a long-term basis. After 5–10 years of treatment there is a slightly increased risk of breast cancer and some women may prefer to stop taking oestrogen after that length of time. They may, however, choose to continue taking oestrogen, bearing in mind its benefits.

It is advisable for a woman to use some form of contraception for at least 12 months after her menopause.

PSYCHOSEXUAL PROBLEMS

Although the exact prevalence of psychosexual problems in men and women is unknown it has been estimated that approximately one-third of women experience sexual difficulties of some kind. The GP should be able to take a relevant history, carry out a pelvic examination, reassure when the findings are normal and be able to refer appropriately either to a gynaecologist or to a psychosexual counsellor when the findings are abnormal.

History

A full case history is essential, with particular emphasis on the problem itself. Patients may complain of any or a combination of the following:

- Apareunia
- Superficial dyspareunia
- Deep dyspareunia
- Decreased libido
- Disparity in libido between the partners
- Lack of self-confidence
- Feelings of inadequacy

Psychosexual problems may occur following pregnancy, the menopause or surgical procedures. Following childbirth a patient may be highly preoccupied with the new child and ignore her partner. Following an induced abortion for an unwanted pregnancy a patient may develop feelings of guilt and these may impact on her sexuality. Following the menopause many women experience superficial dyspareunia due to vaginal dryness and decreased libido. An operation may affect sexual behaviour in several ways.

Following a colostomy a patient may feel 'different' and be unwilling to partake in normal sexual relations – often with the worry that her partner may find her repulsive. Although the operation of abdominal hysterectomy does not compromise the size or function of the vagina some patients may be concerned that their sexuality may be affected. The operation of (simple or radical) vulvectomy with excision of the clitoris has obvious implications for sexual behaviour.

A systemic illness such as diabetes mellitus, hypothyroidism or psychiatric conditions may lead to an overall loss of libido; in some cases the woman is simply too exhausted to have sexual relations.

Pelvic examination
Often a detailed history, a pelvic examination and the confirmation that all is normal are what the patient requires before being reassured that she is 'normal' and being able to return to a satisfying sexual relationship with her partner. A thorough pelvic examination is very important and you should look for the following in particular:

- Vaginismus
- Perineal scarring
- Evidence of previous surgery to the lower genital tract, for example female circumcision
- Evidence of infection of the lower genital tract
- Pelvic endometriosis
- Pelvic tumours
- Pregnancy

Once the pelvic examination is completed it is essential to allow the patient to dress herself and be seated comfortably before the discussion continues.

Management
The general practitioner can play a significant role in reassurance, counselling and education. The discussion must be open and ignorance (if present) must be overcome. A patient with a narrow vagina – for example following vaginal repair operations (see p. 136) – may be given vaginal dilators and instructions on self-application at home. Poor lubrication may be overcome using jellies which are available over the counter. Atrophic vaginitis, however, requires the use of local oestrogen application to the vagina.

You may consider the following for referral to a gynaecologist:

- Presence of perineal/vaginal scarring with tenderness
- Recurrent lower genital tract infection
- Patients suffering from deep dyspareunia
- Patients suspected of suffering from pelvic endometriosis
- Patients suffering from decreased libido despite having an adequate

level of oestrogen replacement therapy – such patients may benefit from a testosterone implant.

A psychosexual counsellor is invaluable in the management of many patients. The presence of the following factors in a patient may indicate referral to a psychosexual counsellor:

- A history of traumatic experience – examples of this include sexual assault and incest
- A history of sexual failure, such as apareunia.
- Absence of risk factors in the case history and normal findings on pelvic examination with persistent symptoms unresponsive to reassurance
- Problems in communicating with partner
- No self-esteem
- Personality disorders

The partner
It should go without saying that an adequate case history should involve details of the patient's partner. The general practitioner should be able to assess information on the partner's age, occupation, state of health, previous medical history, social history and the relationship between the partner and the woman. Among other causes of an unsatisfying sexual relationship, a male partner may suffer from impotence, premature ejaculation, depression and lack of libido. A general practitioner is ideally placed to help a couple with psychosexual problems and often the opening of a channel of communication is therapeutic. It is, however, important to be aware of what problems may be encountered and when to refer the couple to the appropriate specialists.

COUNSELLING

Counselling is made up of three components: the counsellor should *define*, *explore* and *clarify* issues for the patient. The modern doctor works within a team of professionals and so patients are often well informed; it is, however, essential to develop good counselling skills based on a doctor's individual education, training and experience.

The question behind the question
A patient's symptoms, her reaction to them, the result of disability and the expectations for treatment are influenced by various factors. The GP must be aware of the following:

- The patient's illness
- Her perception of her illness
- Family history of the same or similar illness
- The experiences of a close friend or neighbour with the same or similar illness

Many patients are expressive and straightforward in reporting their symptoms and voicing their own concerns. It is, however, useful to have a list of potential concerns that the patient may have. A 'symptom' may be a way of 'breaking the ice' and establishing a channel of communication. Patients may have the following questions in mind when they come to see the general practitioner in the surgery.

- Have I got a form of cancer?
- Have I got venereal disease?
- Am I pregnant?
- Am I infertile?
- Am I feminine?

Requisites for counselling
In order to provide a satisfactory level of counselling you need *all* of the following:

- Time
- The ability to listen
- The ability to sympathetically acknowledge the patient's feelings and concerns (and those of her partner and relatives)
- An appropriate level of knowledge and expertise
- An understanding of the diagnosis
- The ability to be non-judgemental in providing advice
- The capacity to define, explore and clarify without being unduly directional
- Awareness of the availability of local services
- Awareness of the accessibility of regional services

AUDIT

Clinical audit is defined as the critical analysis of the routine care that is given to patients. It is important to distinguish clinical audit from clinical research; research entails *adding* to knowledge, whereas clinical audit is an investigation of what actually happens to patients and related items such as case notes and the results of investigations in everyday practice.

Standards and evidence
Clinical audit involves the examination of accepted or recommended standards, critically investigating processes in patient management in order to see whether the standards have been met or exceeded and making recommendations for change. Standards are set by professional bodies such as the Royal Colleges or by more local institutions. A GP must be able to classify the strength of the evidence which is being used to set the standards. The NHS Executive uses the following system of classification of evidence.

The audit cycle

The audit cycle is represented by Fig. 4.2. A GP may be involved in audit projects at national, regional or local level. The appropriate data are gathered by filling in forms and this body of data are analysed critically. The findings would be compared against the standards which have been set for a certain procedure or process. In effect, the first part of audit compares what actually happened with what *should* have happened. Based on the differences between the standards that have been set and those that have actually been achieved, the next phase in the audit cycle is to recommend changes. The changes should be implemented and the audit cycle completed after an appropriate length of time by a further investigation in order to see whether or not the changes have been implemented and if the standards now achieved were actually the standards that had been set.

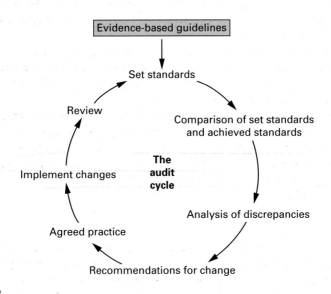

Fig. 4.2

NOTES ON FAMILY PLANNING

5

The main types of contraception are listed below:

- The combined oral contraceptive pill
- The progestogen-only pill
- Post-coital contraception
- Injectable contraceptives
- Intrauterine contraceptive devices
- Barrier methods
- Sterilization

COMBINED ORAL CONTRACEPTION (COC)

The combined oral contraceptive pill (COC) is an effective reversible method of contraception, and with the progestogen-only pill (POP) it is the main method of contraception for 25% of couples in Britain. The POP accounts for about 2.5% of these but between the ages 20–30 up to 50% of all women use the COC.

The COC contains the two synthetic hormones, oestrogen and progestogen. Ethinylestradiol is the usual oestrogen, normally combined with a variety of progestogens including norethisterone, levonorgestrel, desogestrel, gestodene and norgestimate.

Current COCs are either fixed-dose or phasic. The phasic pills are either bi- or triphasic; they still contain oestrogen and progestogen but the dose changes once or twice in the cycle. The phasic pills provide a lower total dose of hormones in the cycle although this has no proven health benefits. Phasic pills are claimed to provide better cycle control. Examples of COCs are given in Table 5.1.

Mode of action

The primary mode of action is prevention of ovulation by lack of follicular maturation and abolition of the oestrogen feedback leading to the LH surge.

In addition, there are cervical mucus changes that reduce sperm penetration and alteration of progesterone receptors which interfere with successful implantation.

Table 5.1   Examples of combined oral contraceptive pills

Type	Pill	(number of tablets)	Oestrogen	Progestogen
Monophasic	Ovysmen		ethinylestradiol 35 μg	norethisterone 0.5 mg
Monophasic	Microgynon		ethinylestradiol 30 μg	levonorgestrel 0.15 mg
Monophasic	Marvelon		ethinylestradiol 30 μg	desogestrel 0.15 mg
Biphasic	BiNovum	(7)	ethinylestradiol 35 μg	norethisterone 0.5 mg
		(14)	ethinylestradiol 35 μg	norethisterone 1.0 mg
Triphasic	Logynon	(5)	ethinylestradiol 30 μg	levonorgestrel 0.05 mg
		(6)	ethinylestradiol 40 μg	levonorgestrel 0.075 mg
		(10)	ethinylestradiol 30 μg	levonorgestrel 0.125 mg

Efficacy

The COC is very effective and completely reversible. Its effectiveness is influenced by compliance, absorption and interaction with other medication. Failure rates per 100 woman years range from 0.2–3 for less than 50 μg pills, and 0.1–3 for 50 μg pills. In the Oxford/FPA study (see p. 177) the overall rate for < 50 μg pills was 0.27, and for 50 μg was 0.16.

Important aspects of counselling

The GP should provide comprehensive instruction on correct usage and starting the pill. In addition, instructions should be given for management of missed pills and the greater significance of this when close to the pill-free week has to be explained. The '7-day rule' advises that if a pill is missed for more than 12 hours take the missed pill immediately and continue other pills as normal but use extra precautions (such as condoms) for the next 7 days. If fewer than 7 pills remain in the pack, the next pack should be started without a break.

You should also advise regarding minor side effects including headaches, weight gain and breakthrough bleeding.

Confirm that there are no contraindications or risk factors (see below) and advise the patient against smoking. Advise sensitively about the associated risk of breast cancer and the pill's protective effects against endometrial and ovarian cancer. Lastly, advice regarding health issues such as genital infection and smears should not be forgotten.

Contraindications for COCs

Some of these contraindications may not be absolute.

Existing cardiovascular disease/thromboembolism.   There is increased risk of venous thromboembolism while taking the COC. The risk appears to be higher in pills containing gestodene and desogestrel. In those who have never used the pill the risk is 5/100 000 women, in gestodene/desogestrel pill users

30/100 000 and in levonorgestrel/norethisterone pill users 15/100 000.

There is no increase in the incidence of ischaemic heart disease (IHD) with use of the COC by non-smokers without hypertension or diabetes. Hypertension, smoking and IHD are separate risk factors for a myocardial infarction and contraindicate the use of the COC.

There is a slight increase in the incidence of ischaemic stroke of approximately 1.5-fold in COC users who are non-smokers and normotensive.

The COC should be avoided if factors exist which predipose to cardiovascular disease such as hypertension, smoking, obesity, diabetes and increased lipids.

Crohn's disease and inflammatory bowel disease may occur more frequently in COC users and because of the increased risk of venous thrombosis when these bowel diseases are active the COC is contraindicated when these disorders are severe. Also remember other chronic diseases predisposing to thrombosis, including rheumatoid arthritis and SLE.

Focal migraine   This is migraine associated with visual, sensory, speech or motor disturbance. There is an increased incidence of ischaemic stroke in COC users which is increased with migraine sufferers. COC is contraindicated with focal migarine, frequent migarine, migraine requiring the use of ergot derivatives, or migraine with any other cardiovascular risk factor.

Major elective surgery   The patient should stop the COC within 2–4 weeks before major surgery and until fully mobile afterwards.

Liver disease   Active liver disease with abnormal liver function, gallstones prior to cholecystectomy and cholestatic jaundice are contraindications.

Oestrogen-dependent tumours   The pill is contraindicated in women with a history of breast cancer. Note the recent evidence indicating a slight increase in incidence of breast cancer with current use. The risk after discontinuing COC use for 10 years returns to the same risk as non-users.

Other contraindications are noted below:

- Existing or possible pregnancy
- Undiagnosed genital tract bleeding
- Patient anxiety despite counselling

Benefits of COC use
Known benefits of COC use are listed below.

- It is a reliable, reversible method, unrelated to intercourse and under the user's control.
- It provides regular, light periods with relief of dysmenorrhoea and pre-menstrual tension.
- The risk of benign breast disease is reduced.

- It reduces the risk of functional ovarian cysts that result from abnormalities in ovulation.
- The pill provides protection against the risk of endometrial and epithelial ovarian cancer.
- Risk of endometriosis is reduced.
- It decreases the risk of anaemia through reduction of menstrual loss.
- It reduces the risk of PID, with a 50% reduction in the risk of admission to hospital. Infection is thought to be in part mediated by the transport of organisms by sperm and the reduction of sperm penetration and effects on tubal function are thought to account for the COC effect on PID.
- Contraceptive effect includes protection against ectopic pregnancy.

Pregnancy and COC

COC inhibits lactation and should not be used if breastfeeding; in such circumstances POP is a suitable hormonal method.

The COC should not be started earlier than 21 days post-partum because of the increased risk of thrombosis with pregnancy. If the risk of thrombosis is considered significant it may be appropriate to delay starting or consider alternative contraception. If started later than 21 days additional contraception is needed for 7 days.

The COC can be started immediately after an early pregnancy loss as there is no increased morbidity.

PROGESTOGEN-ONLY CONTRACEPTION (POP)

Progestogen-only contraceptives contain progestogen only (with no oestrogen, norethisterone, levonorgestrel, ethinodiol diacetate). Their main mode of action is to promote hostile cervical mucus and unreceptive endometrium. Inhibition of ovulation occurs in 15–40% of women using POP.

POP is appropriate for older women, breastfeeding mothers, smokers, patients with a history of thromboembolic disease, or diabetics.

The first pack should commence on the first day of the period (no additional contraception is needed) and continue daily without a break at the same time each day. Efficacy falls if pills are missed or late (> 3 h late). Missed pills should be taken immediately after noticing and normal pill-taking resumed with additional contraception for 7 days.

It is an effective method of contraception when taken correctly and consistently; the overall failure rate is 0.3–4 /100 woman years.

Side effects of POP

- *Menstrual irregularity.* Changes in the menstrual cycle are common and can settle after a few cycles. Amenorrhoea occurs in some, indicating an inhibition of ovulation.

- *Risk of ectopic pregnancy* increases as POP is more effective in preventing intrauterine rather than extrauterine pregnancies.
- *Increased risk of functional ovarian cysts.* These usually resolve spontaneously but serial ultrasound monitoring may be required.
- *Possible association with breast cancer.* Increased risk following use in previous 5 years was reported in 1996 in the Collaborative Group on Hormonal Factors in Breast Cancer Study, but further research is needed.
- Weight gain, breast tenderness, decreased libido, acne and headaches also occur.

POST-COITAL (EMERGENCY) CONTRACEPTION

Emergency methods of contraception include:

- A combined oestrogen–progestogen oral hormonal preparation
- The post-coital insertion of a copper-containing IUCD
- Progestogen-only oral hormonal preparation (unavailable as a licensed product in the UK)

Combined oestrogen–progestogen emergency contraception

This method requires the oral administration of four tablets containing 50 µg ethinylestradiol plus 500 µg norgestrel (equivalent to 250 µg levonorgestrel) and the approved formulation is Schering PC4. Two tablets should be taken within 72 hours of unprotected intercourse and preferably within 24 hours for maximum protection as the failure rate increases as the interval from coitus to treatment increases. The second dose of two tablets should be taken 12 hours after the first.

A pregnancy rate in users has been reported between 1.9% and 5.3%. Effective contraception must be used after the emergency hormonal method as no protection is provided for the remainder of the cycle.

Common side effects include nausea (50%) and vomiting (20%). Intermenstrual bleeding may occur before the next period which may be early or late in approximately 40%.

Intrauterine emergency contraception

With this method a copper-containing IUCD is inserted in the usual way within 5 days (120 hours) of unprotected intercourse at any time of the menstrual cycle. If unprotected intercourse took place more than 5 days earlier an IUCD may be inserted up to 5 days after the estimated earliest day of ovulation. This method provides the greatest protection of currently available emergency contraceptives with a failure rate of less than 0.1%.

Side effects are similar to those previously described for IUCDs. If permanent contraception with an IUCD is not required then it may be removed during the next menses.

Progestogen-only post-coital contraception

This method requires the oral administration of two 750 µg doses of levonorgestrel. The first should be taken within 72 hours of intercourse and the second 12 hours after the first. Levonorgestrel is not currently licensed for emergency contraceptive use in the UK and no appropriate formulation is available but equivalent doses may be achieved with 20 tablets of Neogest, 25 tablets of Microval or 25 tablets Norgeston.

This method compares favourably with the combined preparation with pregnancy rates reported between 0.8% and 1.6%, and nausea and vomiting occurring less frequently with rates of 23% and 6% respectively.

Management and counselling of patients requiring PCC   Check that all the following points are covered when managing and counselling women who need PCC.

- Review the menstrual cycle and estimate date of ovulation.
- Confirm current contraception with timing of all inadequately protected intercourse and calculate the number of hours since first episode
- Identify any contraindications or conditions that require assessment. Absolute contraindications include pregnancy or allergy. Remember liver disease, migraine headaches, significant venous or arterial thrombosis with hormonal methods and the usual IUCD problems.
- Discuss method options, modes of action, failure rates and side effects.
- For hormonal methods explain clearly when pills should be taken and the possible need for a repeat dose of tablets if vomiting occurs within 2 hours of either dose. Indicate that the next period may be delayed and if the next period is atypical then pregnancy needs to be excluded.
- Explain there is a low risk of fetal abnormality with hormonal methods, indicating that the incidence is similar to the 1% incidence of birth defects occurring in the normal population.
- Discuss contraception in the patient's current cycle and provide long-term advice.
- Consider screening for infection if appropriate.
- Arrange follow-up to review treatment, IUCD check or removal, permanent contraception and results of investigations for genitourinary infection.

INJECTABLE CONTRACEPTIVES

There are two injectable contraceptive methods in the UK: Depo-Provera (medroxyprogesterone acetate) and Noristerat (norethisterone enantate).

They act by inhibiting ovulation in addition to increasing cervical mucus hostility and endometrial effects. They are commenced within the first 5 days of menstruation and are immediately effective. Both are given by intramuscular injection. Depo-Provera is given every 12 weeks and

Noristerat every 8 weeks. They are very effective, with failure rates of 0–2/100 woman years.

Side effects
Known side effects of injectable contraceptives include:

- Irregular periods, intermenstrual bleeding or amenorrhoea. Most women experience some menstrual disturbance.
- Secondary amenorrhoea may occur during or after stopping injectable progestogen contraception.
- Other effects include weight gain, headaches, fluid retention, changes in mood and libido, and depression.
- Return to fertility may be delayed by up to a year in some cases.
- There is a possible association with breast cancer but more information is needed.

INTRAUTERINE CONTRACEPTIVE DEVICES (IUCDs)

These are devices which are retained within the uterus for the purpose of preventing contraception. There are four types:

- Inert (no longer available in the UK)
- Copper bearing (Gyne T (discontinued), Nova T, Multiload)
- Hormone releasing (levonorgestrel IUS – Mirena)
- Flexible and frameless (newer devices such as GyneFix)

IUCDs are usually inserted at the end of a period to ensure that the woman is not pregnant and to minimize the risk of expulsion which is higher during menses. They can be inserted up to day 19 of a 28-day cycle (5 days after estimation of ovulation). Modern copper IUCDs have lifespans of 3–10 years.
  Their main mode of action is thought to be prevention of fertilization. All IUCDs cause a foreign body reaction and the inflammatory cells impede sperm transport and fertilization. Sperm phagocytosis has been reported. Copper is also directly toxic to sperm and ova. The progestogen-releasing devices also alter cervical mucus and may inhibit ovulation.
  The overall failure rate is low, with rates from 0.2–2.0/100 woman years. Copper T 380 has a failure rate of 1.4/100 woman years while levonorgestrel IUS is the most effective, with a rate of 0.2/100 woman years.

Side effects and problems
IUCD insertion can have complications including vasovagal episodes, pain and bleeding, infection, perforation and expulsion.
  One of the main problems in using the IUCD can be irregular bleeding or heavier and longer periods.
  There is also an association with pelvic inflamatory disease (PID), and it is generally considered that the overall risk of PID in IUCD users is increased.

This is highest during the first 3 weeks after insertion and the risk of PID is affected by parity, age and sexual activity of the woman and her partner. Perforation is uncommon and occurs in 1/1000 insertions. The risk is increased with puerperal insertion and is common with an inexperienced operator, an unrecognized retroverted uterus or where an instrument is not used to hold the cervix.

The frequency of expulsion varies with a range between 3–15/100 women at 1 year. The risk is greatest during the first 3 months post-insertion and in nulliparous women. Rates decline with age and among IUCD users the expulsion rate is very low after 3 years. Women should be encouraged to check for the IUCD after each period. The GyneFix has the lowest expulsion rate of only 0.4% in the first year.

If threads are missing additional contraception should be used. Pregnancy may also need to be excluded and the woman should be referred for ultrasound to confirm the position of the IUCD and to check for expulsion or perforation. The appropriate management must be arranged.

Extrauterine pregnancies are more common as IUCDs are better at protecting against intrauterine pregnancies. It is important to advise all women to seek medical attention if they develop pelvic pain and menstrual irregularity or amenorrhoea.

Levonorgestrel intrauterine system (IUS)

The IUS is a levonorgestrel-releasing T-shaped device which releases 20 µg/24 h of levonorgestrel from a cylindrical reservoir.

Its mode of action includes endometrial suppression preventing implantation, alteration of cervical mucus, impairment of sperm migration and in some cases inhibition of ovulation. After 1 year 85% have ovulatory cycles. Fertility resumes immediately after removal.

The IUS is a very effective contraceptive with a failure rate of between 0.2 and 0.5/100 woman years.

Menstrual blood flow is reduced significantly and the IUS is therefore effective for the treatment of menorrhagia. It can cause irregular bleeding in the first months after insertion which can take up to 4 months to resolve.

Functional ovarian cysts may occur and are usually asymptomatic but require ultrasound monitoring to confirm spontaneous resolution.

BARRIER METHODS

Female barrier methods include diaphragms, caps and female condoms. They fit into the vagina and cover the cervix thus providing a barrier between the egg and sperm and so preventing fertilization.

Diaphragms are devices with a flexible circular ring covered with latex rubber. They fit into the vagina between the posterior fornix and behind the pubic bone to cover the cervix. *Caps* are smaller than diaphragms and fit directly over the cervix.

Diaphragms have an effectiveness of 1.9/100 woman years (Oxford/FPA study) with a range between 4 and 20/100 woman years. There are no established health risks or systemic side effects with diaphragms and they may protect against cancer of the cervix and PID. The method is directly under the control of the woman and can be inserted prior to intercourse. It must be used with a spermicide. It requires initial fitting by a trained doctor or nurse, and the patient must be taught its correct use. It should be replaced annually and reassessed for size after delivery or miscarriage.

The diaphragm or cap can be fitted at any time before having sex but if inserted more than 3 hours before intercourse additional spermicide should be used. It must be left in place for at least 6 hours after intercourse and usually removed before 30 hours.

Irritation due to sensitivity has been reported. Urethritis may occur more frequently in some users as a result of pressure and require the fitting of a smaller device. Several cases of toxic shock syndrome have been reported in users wearing a diaphragm for more than 30 hours.

The female condom is a single-size lubricated loose-fitting polyurethane sheath with two flexible rings which is inserted into the vagina covering the vaginal walls and vulva. It must be inserted prior to intercourse and used only once. It acts as a contraceptive and protects against sexually transmitted infections. Currently Femidom is the only female condom available in the UK.

Male condoms are made of natural latex or polyurethane. They are worn over the erect penis and provide a barrier between egg and sperm thus preventing fertilization.

Condoms are effective in preventing pregnancy and sexually transmitted infections including HIV. They have a failure rate of 3.6/100 woman years (Oxford/FPA study) and a reported range from 2 to 15/100 woman years. They may protect the female partner against cancer of the cervix.

STERILIZATION

Female sterilization can be performed at laparoscopy, laparotomy or at the time of Caesarean section. The method of choice in the UK is laparoscopy for access to the Fallopian tubes and mechanical occlusion with either clips or rings. A laparotomy may be more appropriate if there is a relevant past history of abdominopelvic surgery, adhesions, or in patients with obesity.

The tubes can be occluded using Falope rings, Filshie clips or by tubal destruction using diathermy or by other techniques involving ligation and excision of a section of tube (Pomeroy).

Sterilization is usually performed as a day-case procedure under general anaesthesia although local anaesthesia is an acceptable alternative. The operation can be performed at any time during the menstrual cycle but contraception should be continued until the next menses following the procedure.

Vasectomy (male sterilization) should include division of each vas deferens or removal of a piece of each vas, in either case accompanied by fascial interposition or diathermy.

The procedure is usually performed under local anaesthesia and the vas is accessed by single or bilateral scrotal incisions.

Effectiveness

Female sterilization is effective with a lifetime failure rate of approximately 1/200. The risk of failure varies by procedure, method and age. Male sterilization is more effective than female with a lifetime failure rate of 1/2000 following two azoospermic samples. The Oxford /FPA study reports failure rates per 100 woman years for female sterilization of 0.13 and male sterilization of 0.02.

Side effects

Menstrual disturbance has been reported but this may be related to age, stopping the COC, or other gynaecological problems. If pregnancy occurs the risk of ectopic pregnancy is higher. Psychological problems or regret are more common in those under the age of 25 years or in those patients without children. Sexual activity and enjoyment should be unaffected.

Male sexual libido and functioning should be unaffected. Short-term effects after vasectomy include bruising and swelling which may last a couple of weeks. Scrotal haematoma occurs in 6%, and sperm granuloma may cause a foreign body reaction with discrete tender nodules in 30% which may require excision. Sperm antibodies occur in 60–80% of men following vasectomy and do not cause any health problems but the antibodies can reduce the pregnancy success rate after reversal of vasectomy. There is no increased risk of cardiovascular disease, testicular or prostate cancer after vasectomy.

Counselling and consent issues

Careful and thorough counselling is essential prior to sterilization. All the issues raised below should be covered with couples seeking sterilization.

- Confirm awareness of alternative methods of long-term contraception. Both vasectomy and tubal occlusion should always be discussed and both the lower failure rate and lower procedure-associated risks with vasectomy should be emphasized.
- If appropriate, indicate the increased incidence of regret associated with those under 25 years or without children and the increased risk of regret and possible increased failure rate if tubal occlusion is performed post-pregnancy.
- Clarify that the sterilization procedure is permanent.

- The risk of pregnancy following the procedure needs to be clearly explained. In women it is approximately 1/200 and in men 1/2000 after two azoospermic samples 2–4 weeks apart at least 8 weeks after the procedure.
- Women should be warned of the increased risk of ectopic pregnancy, which may be a fatal condition.
- The method of sterilization should be clearly explained including the risks associated with surgery and the possibility of needing a laparotomy during a laparoscopic procedure.
- Women should also be advised that they must use effective contraception prior to sterilization and continue until their next period after the procedure.
- Men need effective contraception until two consecutive semen samples confirm azoospermia 2–4 weeks apart.
- Reassure couples that there are no serious long-term health risks associated with sterilization procedures.

REFERENCES

1. Belfield, T. (1999) *FPA Contraceptive Handbook* (3rd edn)., Family Planning Association, London.
2. Loudon, N. B., Glasier, A., Gebbie, A. (1995) *Handbook of Family Planning and Reproductive Health Care* (3rd edn). Churchill Livingstone, Edinburgh.
3. Guillebaud, J. (1993) *Contraception: Your Questions Answered* (2nd edn). Churchill Livingstone, Edinburgh.
4. RCOG Guidelines no 4 (1994 and 1997) *Male and Female Sterilization.* RCOG, London.
5. Collaborative Group on Hormonal Factors in Breast Cancer (1996) *Lancet*, 347, 1713–1727.
6. Oxford/FPA Contraceptive Study (1982) *Lancet*, 1, 841–2.

NOTES ON OBSTETRICS

6

PREGNANCY – GENERAL NOTES

Physiological changes in pregnancy
The uterus stretches and hypertrophies without new cell development due to hormonal change, mainly oestrogen and progesterone, both of which initiate changes in the uterine musculature at the beginning of the second trimester. After that time there is a direct stretching activity of the uterine muscle. Corpus luteum of the ovary is the source of progesterone, which maintains the pregnancy during the first 7 weeks; after that time the placenta takes over the role of producing progesterone.

There are many other changes associated with pregnancy. In the pulmonary system, for example, there is mild compensated respiratory alkalosis. In the cardiovascular system a hyper-dynamic state is caused by a 50% increase in the bloodflow. This results in the increased resting pulse, cardiac output and the flow murmurs that are associated with pregnancy. There is also a progressive decrease in peripheral vascular resistance and this will lead to the slight decrease in blood pressure noted in normal second trimester.

Supine hypotensive syndrome of pregnancy arises due to the compression of the interior vena cava by the enlarged uterus when the pregnant woman is lying supine, and this can significantly decrease the venous blood return to the heart; subsequently, maternal dizziness upon rising can occur. In extreme cases this syndrome can cause fetal distress.

In a normal pregnancy there are certain physiological changes, for example haemodilutional anaemia and ureteric dilatation, especially on the right side. This may be due to a progesterone effect caused by mechanical compression of the enlarged uterus.

Glycosuria may also be seen in a normal pregnancy due to an increased glomerular filtration rate. As regards the gastrointestinal tract there is a delayed gastric emptying time, the oesophageal sphincter tone becomes poor, there is an increase in the volume of the gall bladder and the motility of the gastrointestinal tract decreases.

Carpal tunnel syndrome, bilaterally or unilaterally, may arise during pregnancy. This may be due to fluid retention and compression of the radial nerve on the flexor retinaculum. In about 10–15% of cases of carpal tunnel syndrome, surgery may be required during pregnancy to relieve severe pain.

The incidence of Bell's palsy increases in pregnancy due to unilateral facial nerve palsy with upper and lower facial involvement. Conservative management is all that is needed.

The fetal heart beats by day 22 and may be detected on ultrasound scan within 6–7 weeks. The fetus has a higher serum haemoglobin than the adult, about 18 g/dl compared with 13 g/dl.

DIAGNOSIS OF PREGNANCY

Symptoms of pregnancy include amenorrhoea, nausea, vomiting, breast changes and urinary symptoms.

The signs of pregnancy include characteristic changes in the breast and uterus.

The investigations include a variety of pregnancy tests including tests for beta sub-unit human chorionic gonadotrophin (see Chapter 4). Modern tests can detect human chorionic gonadotrophin before the time of the missed period.The monoclonal antibody test for HCG and beta sub-units are sensitive and specific of pregnancy. The enzyme-linked immunosorbent assays (ELISA) give positive results at much lower levels of human chorionic gonadotrophin and so can be positive very early in the pregnancy.

Ultrasound has also made a remarkable improvement to the diagnosis of pregnancy. With modern machines and vaginal probes, pregnancy can be diagnosed very early; the fetal heart can be detected at 6 weeks using the vaginal probe and at 7 weeks using the transabdominal probe.

ANTENATAL CARE

The time at which a woman is usually seen for booking at her hospital varies from one hospital to another but ideally this is done between 8–10 weeks' gestation; more frequently, the history is taken in the community.

The points to be elaborated in the history on the first visit include previous or current maternal diseases, in particular hypertensive disease, diabetes, endocrine diseases and liver disorders. The family history should include significant diseases among blood relatives. It is also important to establish the date of the last normal menstrual period and the pattern of periods; and if the woman is sure of her dates. It is essential to elaborate on the cycle pattern and whether or not the woman was taking the contraceptive pill.

It is also important to establish whether the pregnancy was planned or not.

To calculate the expected date of confinement confirm the date of the first day of the last normal menstrual period, deduct 3 months and add 7 days.

This rule applies only to women with a regular cycle and those who have stopped oral contraceptives or any form of contraception at least a couple of months before the last few normal periods. If in doubt about the dates, because of uncertainty as to the time of the last period, a dating scan is now available and the GP can arrange this through most hospitals.

It is important also to take a history of smoking at the time of booking and *advise against it.*

In an ideal world women with existing health problems should have been seen in the pre-conception clinic if there is a consultant obstetrician who is interested in this.

Alternatively, if you feel that your patient needs pre-conception counselling, this can be arranged with the consultant with whom you are going to share the care of the pregnant woman.

General examination is of paramount importance in the booking visit in that it may be the first medical examination for several years; recording of the booking blood pressure and weight, listening to the heart and lungs, and palpation of the breasts and abdomen are its principal components. The fetal heart can be auscultated from 12 weeks with modern fetal heart detectors, but always explain to the patient that it may not be possible to hear the fetal heart at 12 weeks so she should not be anxious if you fail to demonstrate the baby's heart rate.

Pelvic examination is unnecessary at booking although some gynaecologists still perform it as a routine and obtain a cervical smear if the woman has had no smear in the past.

Antenatal visits generally take place every 4 weeks until 28 weeks and then every 2 weeks until 36 weeks and weekly thereafter. The frequency of antenatal visits for 'low-risk' women has been extensively reviewed since the published findings of the Audit Commission in 1997. The community midwife can deal with most of these visits in the surgery.

Most hospitals see the pregnant woman at booking, at 36 weeks and after that at 41 weeks but this must be checked with the policy of the local hospital; plan the visits at your surgery and with the community midwife accordingly.

Routine investigations at booking include a full blood count, urine analysis, blood grouping and Rh factor, antibodies to Rh factor if Rh negative, serological tests for syphilis, rubella and maternal serum alpha fetoprotein.

In certain ethnic groups testing for sickle-cell disease and other haemoglobin abnormalities is required. Similarly in the 'at risk' population, screening for chlamydial infections, hepatitis and even HIV should be performed with the patient's permission. Screening for hepatitis B is now offered routinely. Some units perform alpha fetoprotein (AFP) screening as a routine plus other investigations depending on the population in their area. The test is very sensitive to gestational age, therefore accurate dating is required. An early dating scan is of great help. A high serum AFP expressed as multiples of the median (MOM) usually means that the woman should be offered a high-resolution ultrasound scan to exclude open neural tube defects having excluded missed abortion, twins and miscalculated gestation. A detailed scan is usually performed between 19–20 weeks in most hospitals. The reason for this is the ability to demonstrate any heart problems at this stage.

Radiographers usually perform the ultrasound scan and after the detection or suspicions of any abnormalities a radiologist or obstetrician with a special interest in ultrasound has to confirm the findings and counsel the pregnant woman accordingly. There are many ultrasound markers that point to fetal chromosomal abnormality and the standard antenatal scan at 19–20 weeks includes a careful search for such signs.

At 28, 32 and 36 weeks there is a need to check for antibodies in Rh negative women. This does not necessarily have to be performed in hospital and can be carried out at the surgery or by the community midwife.

General advice to pregnant women
At booking there is a great opportunity to prepare the mother-to-be, and advising her to stop or reduce smoking is very important. Advice on alcohol consumption should similarly be offered. Advice should also be given about a good balanced diet, exercise, rest and suitable clothing.

Some women may need to be advised about the safety of intercourse during pregnancy and be reassured that it has no harmful effects.

Assessment of fetus during pregnancy
Assessment of the growing fetus is of paramount importance. Most pregnancies progress normally and the aim of the antenatal check-up is to detect and treat any abnormalities.

There are various methods of assessment, but basically the clinical assessment is traditional and very effective in experienced hands. Fetal growth should be checked regularly. We have to accept that although clinical assessment is rather a crude method, even in the best hands, it enables the recognition of problems and investigations can be initiated. Maternal assessment should be undertaken at the same time.

Other methods of assessing fetal wellbeing include biophysical profile, cardiotocography (CTG) and Doppler studies of the fetus.

Biophysical profile
The introduction of ultrasound has added to the methods of assessing the fetus in utero. The biophysical profile includes assessment of fetal tone, fetal movement, the amniotic fluid volume, the assessment of the fetal breathing movements and interpretation of the cardiotocograph (CTG).

It is essential to note that each of these tests has a false positive rate of about 20%. They are time consuming and should be reserved for the 'at risk' group of obstetric patients.

Ultrasound in early pregnancy

Ultrasound has had an important impact on obstetrics in general. There are three levels of ultrasound scanning in pregnancy: the first level detects the viability of the pregnancy and the number of fetuses; the second level is normally carried out at 18–20 weeks to detect any abnormality; the third level is performed in special referral centres with clinicians who are specialized in fetal medicine.

Measurement of biparietal diameter (BPD) and the fetal femur length are used to establish accurate gestational age. Assessment of fetal growth is achieved by measuring the fetal head circumference and abdominal circumference.

Ultrasound may also be used as a method for detecting small-for-dates or growth retarded fetuses by performing serial measurements of fetal growth.

Nutrition in pregnancy

An ideal pre-pregnancy body weight is important but this is difficult to achieve for many women. For example, if a pre-pregnant weight is less than 80% of an ideal body weight, the woman is at risk of having a baby with a low birth weight (less than 2.5 kg). It has been recognized that improving nutrition in pregnancy can significantly improve the birth weight of infants. Dietary counselling is, therefore, important and should be offered prior to pregnancy. In any case advice on balanced nutrition is of paramount importance at the booking unit.

Special consideration should be given to an obese woman, although it is important to identify the fact that pregnancy is not the right time to diet. A dietician should be involved if necessary.

Some women are very worried about a poor weight increase in pregnancy and this group should be reassured. The basic nutritional requirement for a pregnant woman is a sensible diet derived from protein, fruits, vegetables, carbohydrates and an appropriate level of fat.

Adequate nutrition is difficult to maintain in those who may present with severe morning sickness. Here the advice is to have small and frequent meals without liquids, although liquids should be encouraged between meals.

Oral iron supplement is given as a routine in some units but folic acid is an essential supplement that should always be given as a routine.

There are certain types of food which are not recommended for pregnant women, but overall a well-balanced diet should be advised.

Activity in pregnancy

Pregnant women should be encouraged to take routine exercise, such as swimming, walking and mild exercise, as these should not affect pregnancy. High-impact aerobic exercises are best avoided as injuries may occur. Skiing and gymnastics should be advised against in pregnancy.

Symptoms of pregnancy

Nausea is common in the early weeks of pregnancy, usually in the morning, and improves at approximately 14 weeks. No drugs are needed. For severe nausea and vomiting, anti-histamines may sometimes be given. A common and safe drug is cyclizine. Admission to hospital occasionally proves necessary.

Heartburn is common in pregnancy due to the physiological relaxation of the oesophagus and pyloric sphincters, resulting in reflux of bile and acid. Progesterone and the pressure from the uterus are additional factors for delayed gastric emptying. Treatment is usually symptomatic and antacids can be used.

Oedema of the legs is rather common in pregnancy due to fluid retention and venous obstruction resulting from the pressure of the gravid uterus. Elevation of the legs usually reduces the swelling. Diuretics should not be given to treat oedema of pregnancy.

Constipation affects 20–30% of pregnant women. Advice regarding diet is all that is needed.

If a physiological discharge per vagina is noticed in pregnancy reassurance and advice are all that are needed.

Breathlessness occurs in about 30–50% of pregnant women and is most likely to be due to hyperventilation of pregnancy and increase in the cardiac output. Having excluded major pathological causes of breathlessness such as anaemia or heart and lung disease, reassurance is all that is needed.

Some pregnant women develop exaggerated lumbar lordosis and strain, suffering backache. Advice is all that is needed and sometimes a mild form of analgesics may be used.

Haemorrhoids may occur during pregnancy, aggravated by constipation. Conservative treatment is helpful. A surgical opinion may be needed in severe cases of haemorrhoids.

Headache is a rather difficult symptom of pregnancy, which may be aggravated by constipation. You should enquire whether the woman has a history of migraine and she should be treated with paracetamol. It is always useful to check on the vision of the pregnant woman as some may suffer from headaches due to a cause which preceded the pregnancy.

A dental check is also advisable – pregnant women have free services.

Itching is a rare symptom. If it occurs and is alarming, liver function tests should be checked to exclude cholestasis of pregnancy which may present with recurrent jaundice.

There are many other symptoms which may and do occur in pregnant women. Reassurance is all that is essential as part of the treatment, especially in the primigravida.

BLEEDING IN PREGNANCY

This is a major concern for the woman, her family and the GP. The clinical significance increases with the progress of pregnancy and it may cause maternal morbidity and/or mortality. Assess gestational age and viability.

Bleeding in early pregnancy

About 80% of spontaneous pregnancy losses occur in the first trimester. Within 20 weeks' gestation, 15–20% of recognized pregnancies are complicated by bleeding and more than half of these will end in miscarriage. The risk of spontaneous miscarriage increases with advanced maternal age.

Diagnosis and management

A normal pregnancy can be visualized by vaginal ultrasound when the sac diameter is more than 4 mm. The heart starts to beat on day 22–23 of fetal life and can be detected at around $5\frac{1}{2}$ to 6 weeks.

An anembryonic pregnancy is defined as an intrauterine sac without fetal tissue at a gestation of more than $7\frac{1}{2}$ weeks. When the diameter of the sac is 16 mm or more and there is no visible embryo, this is defined as non-viable in all cases.

Delayed miscarriage may be managed medically with a combination of mifepristone and prostaglandin analogue. This, of course, can be offered to women with delayed miscarriage who are reluctant to have surgical evacuation. In some cases they need surgical evacuation, however, and that should be done carefully as complications may arise in such patients.

Bleeding in late pregnancy

This is a common cause of perinatal mortality and morbidity in the developing countries. Any pregnant woman with bleeding in late pregnancy should be assessed carefully. Antepartum haemorrhage (APH) has traditionally been defined as vaginal bleeding after a gestation age of 28 weeks, but with improvements in neonatal intensive care, the survival rate has improved. Viability has been reduced to 22 weeks in some countries. In the UK, the threshold for viability is 24 weeks. In practice it is wise to consult the delivery suite if a patient needs admission.

Known causes of bleeding in late pregnancy include: abruptio placentae, placenta praevia, vasa praevia, other local causes, haematuria which should be identified and excluded, and cervical problems including cancer and rectal bleeding.

Abruptio placentae

The term describes bleeding from a normally situated placenta, which may be either a revealed, concealed or mixed haemorrhage. It is associated with pre-eclampsia, poor nutrition, high parity, polyhydramnios, external cephalic version and previous history of abruption. Recurrence is about 16% after one and about 20% after two previous abruptions.

Abruptio placentae is associated with both maternal and fetal risks. It presents as severe constant pain, which may or may not be associated with vaginal bleeding. The degree of shock in this condition is out of proportion to the extent of blood loss. The uterus is tender and there is difficulty in feeling it.

Renal involvement and disseminated intravascular coagulation (DIC) may develop.

Acute surgical conditions, rectus sheath haematoma, uterine rupture and degeneration of uterine fibroid are to be remembered as differential diagnoses for abruption.

Management   Prevention is impossible as there is no known cause for abruption but there are associated factors. Chronic hypertension, severe pre-eclampsia, previous abruption, pre-term labour, pre-term rupture of membranes and abdominal trauma seem to be the strongest risk factors associated with abruption.

The patient should be informed about the risk that bleeding could continue. She may suffer continuous abdominal pain, sudden onset of contractions, reduced fetal movements and on some occasions the loss of the fetus.

The fetal heart should be monitored continuously or frequently depending on the clinical condition. A soft abdomen on palpation and a normal fetal heart can almost certainly exclude cases of massive abruption. The pregnancy could, therefore, be allowed to continue unless the patient is near term, when induction of labour may be considered in some cases.

Amniotomy is the method of choice for induction as it lowers intraamniotic pressure and therefore reduces the amount of thromboplastin being released into the circulation.

If the cervix is unfavourable for amniotomy to be performed, give prostaglandin to induce uterine contractions and wait for the cervix to be more favourable. The uterus is more prone to rupture in patients with abruptio placentae.

If the cervix is unfavourable you could wait for a few hours for the dilatation to occur with Prostin. When cervical change starts, progress is usually very rapid.

Provided the patient's condition remains stable and there is no severe haemorrhage slow progress is not a major problem. Urine output should be observed closely and so should the platelet count which should be carried out every 4–6 hours.

A low platelet count indicates possible intravascular coagulation; regular coagulation studies until after delivery are therefore indicated.

In cases of a smaller abruption with a stable maternal condition and no fetal distress, expectant treatment is usually beneficial and it may allow the pregnancy to continue further.

Management of abruption with confirmed intrauterine fetal death implies that the size of abruption was large. In these cases coagulation deficiency is found in about 60% of cases. The patients are usually hypovolaemic owing to the blood loss, which may be totally *concealed*: fluid should be replaced with crystalloid solution and blood and further replacement of fluid depends on the renal output. Examine the cervix, and if it is favourable and the membranes are well formed they should be ruptured to start contractions and reduce the intrauterine pressure.

Unless labour proceeds quickly prompt action will be required to prevent further complications.

Placenta praevia

This refers to location of the placenta over or within the internal os. Traditionally it has been classified in four degrees as outlined in Box 6.1.

Box 6.1 Degrees of placenta praevia

Grade 1   The placenta encroaches the lower uterine segment but not close to the cervical os

Grade 2   The placenta is implanted in the lower uterine segment, coming close to the internal os of the cervix

Grade 3   The internal os is partially covered by the placenta

Grade 4   The internal os is completely covered by the placenta

---

The incidence of placenta praevia is less than 1% of all deliveries, and the aetiology is unknown. It occurs usually in older women and those who have had previous Caesarean sections. With the development of ultrasound, the diagnosis of placenta praevia is easy and accurate in pregnancy. However, in early pregnancy when the lower segment has not developed the placenta may lie near the internal os but appears to migrate as the lower segment develops.

Prior to the development of ultrasound, examination under anaesthesia was the popular method of establishing the position of the placenta. This is rarely needed in modern obstetric practice.

Management   Management of a woman with placenta praevia depends on the stage of pregnancy and the grade. Between 24–34 weeks all patients with a major placenta praevia should be admitted to hospital from around 26 weeks to 30 weeks. Repeated bleeding even with minor loss necessitates urgent delivery. Bed-rest is recommended as this may reduce uterine activity after stretching of the lower segment and the subsequent detachment of the placenta.

Care should be taken that the serum Hb does not drop below 11 g/dl as this lowers the patient's reserve in case of severe haemorrhage. Steroids should be given prior to 30 weeks to enhance lung maturity.

In late pregnancy, between 34–37 weeks, management is similar but steroids are no longer needed. At term, if the head is engaged a senior obstetrician should assess the patient and decide the mode of delivery: if the patient is to have a Caesarean section, this should again be carried out by a senior obstetrician; operative delivery carries the risk of *severe* haemorrhage and this is why the surgeon must be experienced and blood must be available for possible transfusion.

For the inexperienced surgeon a vertical abdominal incision is preferred as it gives better exposure under difficult conditions.

Large veins may overlie the lower segment and should be tied before the uterine incision is made.

In pre-term pregnancies the lower segment may be poorly developed, and especially when the head is high or the presentation is breech it may be extremely difficult to deliver the fetus through the narrow lower segment and here a vertical incision may be preferred. Severe haemorrhage may obscure the surgeon's view immediately after delivery of the placenta. This usually comes from the lower segment of the uterus, which is known not to contract effectively to control bleeding. Bleeding is usually of venous origin and it may best be controlled by temporarily applied pressure. Arterial bleeding points should be clamped and ligated.

After the removal of the placenta, bleeding from vessels is minimal but the remaining bleeders are usually few and they may be controlled with repeated figure-of-8 sutures.

These details may not be relevant for your practice as a general practitioner, but it is important to be aware of them for counselling and explanation to your patients.

Local causes of antepartum haemorrhage
The most common cause is ectopy of the cervix, as the cervix becomes very vascular during pregnancy. Another local cause is carcinoma of the cervix, which occurs rather frequently and early in some populations. Speculum examination is therefore essential in order not to miss such an important diagnosis. Before examining any pregnant woman with vaginal bleeding, check placental location.

APH of unknown origin   Patients in this category should be carefully monitored in hospital for the first 24 h after admission. Before discharge from hospital the cervix should be examined digitally.

HYPERTENSION IN PREGNANCY

Hypertension in pregnancy is defined as two consecutive readings of 140/90 mmHg or above. Readings should be at least 4 hours apart. A rise in blood pressure over a booking value of > 30 point systolic or > 15 point diastolic is an appropriate definition. Always check the booking blood pressure.

The reported incidence of hypertension in pregnancy is about 5–7% of all pregnancies. About 1% of all pregnant women will present with a blood pressure of 170/110 mmHg.

According to recent confidential enquiries, hypertensive disorders in pregnancy are one of the major causes of maternal morbidity and mortality.

Blood pressure should be checked in a semi-recumbent position to avoid pressure on the vena cava and the cuff should be wound at the level of the patient's heart. Remember a large cuff for a large patient (arm circumference > 35 cm). Korokoff Phase IV (the muffling phase) has been used traditionally, but recent evidence recommends phase V (disappearance phase).

There is no universally accepted classification of hypertension in pregnancy. A logical distinction is between pre-pregnancy hypertension and pregnancy-induced hypertension. The pre-existing hypertension may have a number of causes including renal disease, phaeochromocytoma, systemic lupus erythematosus (SLE) and coarctation of the aorta. Pregnancy-induced hypertension (PIH) maybe classified into proteinuric pre-eclampsia and non-proteinuric hypertension.

Mild to moderate PIH is more common in primigravida, aged less than 20 years or more than 35 years. A family history of hypertension, PET (pre-eclamptic toraemia) or maternal eclampsia is known to increase the risk by a factor of 8. Migraine and low body mass are known associated risk factors for mild or moderate PIH.

Moderate to severe PIH is known to be commoner in women with SLE, chronic renal problems, diabetes and women with essential hypertension. Fetal risk factors include molar pregnancy, a large placenta, triploidy and trisomy 13 and 18. Control of pre-existing essential hypertension is known to reduce the risk of severe hypertension. Methyldopa, nifedipine, oxprenolol and labetalol are in use. Remember atenolol has been associated with intrauterine growth retardation.

PET (pre-eclampsia)

This is a multi-system disorder, involving renal and cardiovascular organs and clotting. It is likely to be an immunological disorder.

There is a failure of the normal trophoblastic invasion of the uterine spiral arteries. This process normally removes the muscular component of the walls of the spiral arteries. Trophoblastic embolization increases, which may be the source of the disseminated intravascular coagulation, together with failure of the normal increase in plasma volume.

There is also a reduction in prostacycline – ultimately there are cardiac, brain and renal effects. An increased risk of pulmonary oedema exists. The fetal effects include IUGR, FDIU and iatrogenic prematurity.

Although published evidence does *not* support prophylactic low-dose aspirin, it is still used on an individual basis for those women with a history of an early onset of PET. Aspirin and steroids are used for prophylaxis for patients with SLE although there is some debate about their value. The GP must refer any patient suspected of having PET to a specialist on an emergency basis.

Management of PET   Ultimate treatment is by removing the placenta. Other strategies include monitoring and treating the blood pressure, monitoring proteinuria, fluid balance, uric acid and platelets.

Watch for signs and symptoms of deterioration: headache, epigastric pain, flashing lights.

Monitor fetal growth and wellbeing, and decide the appropriate time for delivery.

Fulminating PET   Note the following strategies:

- Control blood pressure
- Prevent fits
- Monitor fluid balance
- Monitor clotting
- Plan delivery
- Consider magnesium sulfate, phenytoin, diazepam and clomethiazole
- Consider nifedipine, Apresoline and other medications.

HELLP syndrome   This stands for haemolysis (H), elevated liver enzymes (EL) and low platelets (LP). It is a part of severe PET but can occur with relatively mild or moderate hypertension and may not present until after the delivery. It is thought to complicate about 10% of all cases of severe PET; there is evidence that the incidence is rising but this may be due to improved methods of diagnosis.

Management is principally delivery, control of hypertension plus supportive measures until the condition reverses, which it usually does within 48 h of the delivery. Careful fluid balance is vital; platelet transfusions may be needed. If renal failure occurs dialysis will be necessary until normal function returns.

CONGENITAL ABNORMALITIES

The percentage of newborns with a single minor malformation, which may not be quite obvious and has very little effect if any on development, is not known. Multiple pregnancy is associated with a higher incidence of fetal abnormalities than singletons. The overall perinatal mortality from malformation is about 2.5 per 1000 total births. Most congenital defects arise *de novo* and about 20% have multi-factorial reasons. It is interesting to note that chromosomal anomalies account for only about 5% of the total incidence while infections cause about 2% of the total incidence.

Chromosomal abnormality

Most of the fetuses with chromosomal abnormalities are not viable and they could have aneuploidy or polyploidy.

Down's syndrome

Overall, the incidence is about 1/700 live births and 60–80% of affected pregnancies result in miscarriage or stillbirth. The majority are due to trisomy 21 resulting from non-dysjunction during gametogenesis.

At a maternal age of 20 the risk of Down's syndrome is about 1/1530; this rises to 1/37 when the woman is 44. It is important as a GP to counsel women with an affected child that the risk of recurrence of Down's syndrome due to trisomy 21 is about 1 in 100.

Babies with Down's syndrome are usually small for dates and hypotonic. There is a characteristic mongoloid facial feature. The children are usually happy and affectionate with a mean IQ of about 50. It has been observed that many Down's syndrome individuals will develop Alzheimer's disease later in their lives.

The screening for Down's syndrome is usually with biochemical methods or ultrasound scanning. Nuchal fold thickness at around 11–13 weeks is now an established method for screening.

Cystic fibrosis (CF)

This is the commonest chromosomal recessive condition in the UK and 1 in 22 persons are carriers. The CF gene is located on chromosome 7.

The child usually presents with failure to thrive, recurrent chest problems and/or malabsorption. The fetus or the neonate may present with peritoneal calcification or meconium ileus. Pre-term delivery is common and affected mothers are at risk of cardiorespiratory problems and pregnancy should be avoided if possible. Counselling is therefore mandatory.

Adult people with this condition usually suffer from sub-fertility problems.

Haematological problems

Sickle-cell disease   This is commoner in certain racial groups, especially in tropical African countries and among North American blacks, It is caused by alteration in the structure of the globin chains. Heterozygotes are usually protected against *Falciparum* malaria.

Thalassaemia   This may be classified as alpha or beta; homozygous thalassaemia major is usually fatal. Heterozygous thalassaemia minor is the commonest form. Diagnosis is usually suspected in women of Mediterranean origin, although the disease is common in the Far East and Middle East as well. Electrophoresis usually confirms the diagnosis and there is an associated mild anaemia. The spleen is sometimes slightly enlarged with mild jaundice.

The red-blood cell fragility is increased with a low Hb. The serum iron is raised and therefore patients usually require folate supplement. Watch for a haemolytic crisis, which will need admission. Stress and infections should be treated as early as possible.

Neural tube defects
These are by far the commonest anomalies, and the development of ultrasound has had a great impact on early diagnosis. Anencephaly and spina bifida comprise more than 95% of neural tube defects. The incidence is inversely related to socio-economic class and there is definite geographical variation.

The risk for recurrence after one affected child is 1/25, rising to 1/10 after two or more affected children. An affected parent has a 1/25 risk of producing a child with a neural tube defect. The serum alpha fetoprotein may detect up to 90% of anencephaly, 50% of cases of open spina bifida but includes 3% of unaffected singleton pregnancies.

The high resolution ultrasound scan has changed the methods of screening for a neural tube defect.

Pre-pregnancy folic acid in a dose of 400 µg daily taken for at least 1 month before conception and up to about 14 weeks of pregnancy is recommended for the primary prevention of neural tube defects.

Abdominal wall defects
The incidence is about 1/6000 pregnancies. There are two types:

Gastroschisis is identified when the umbilical cord is not involved and there is no sac. There is associated gut atresia and cardiac lesion in about 20%. Ultrasound diagnosis is possible in early pregnancy and maternal serum alpha fetoprotein may be elevated. Isolated defects are amenable to surgical correction.

Exomphalos is identified when the umbilical cord is involved and is attached to the apex of the sac, which in some cases may contain the liver and/or intestines. There is an associated risk of chromosomal anomalies in about 30% of cases and heart lesions in about 10%.

Vaginal delivery is not contraindicated except for obstetric indications.

Congenital heart lesions
The overall incidence of these has increased in recent years to 8 per 1000 births. Pre-natal diagnosis of some of the more serious of the defects is possible by using the high resolution ultrasound scan at around 20–22 weeks' gestation.

Cleft lip and palate
Cleft lip and/or palate occurs in 1/1000 births, mostly multi-factorial in origin. There is an association with more than 100 rare chromosomal

abnormalities or single gene traits. There is a recurrence of about 1/50 if a child presents with unilateral cleft lip and he or she was born to normal parents. This recurrence is about 1/20 if the child was born with bilateral cleft lip and palate to normal parents. The isolated cleft palate is rather different, in that it affects 1/2500 births with a recurrence risk of 1/60 for sibs and offspring. Counselling is therefore essential and an early referral to a geneticist is advisable.

DIAGNOSIS OF CONGENITAL ABNORMALITIES

Ultrasound has become the main diagnostic technique for pre-natal diagnosis. The commonest time for routine examination is between 18–20 weeks. Some techniques should only be carried out in regional tertiary referral centres.

Chorionic villus biopsy (CVB)
The biopsy obtains placental tissue from the chorion under guidance using an ultrasound machine.

The procedure may be transcervical or transabdominal: transcervical CVB can be carried out between 7–10 weeks, whereas transabdominal CVB can be from 8 weeks to term. The additional procedure-related risk of miscarriage is about 2%.

The advantages of this procedure are that it can be carried out early in the first trimester; the tissues are suitable for DNA analysis and the results are available within 48 h.

There is, however, an association with limb defects secondary to trauma at the time of the procedure.

Fetal blood sampling
A sample of fetal blood can be obtained by cordocentesis for diagnostic purposes and this procedure is carried out in special centres.

Other advanced procedures include embryo biopsy and fetal therapy, which are restricted to tertiary referral centres.

Amniocentesis
This is the most commonly performed pre-natal diagnostic test. It is performed from 14 weeks of pregnancy, and karyotype results are normally available within 3 weeks of the procedure.

There is a failure rate with cell culture and the patient should therefore be informed of this.

There is also a risk of miscarriage, which depends on the experience of the operator and varies between 1/100 to 1/200.

The test is done under direct ultrasound and no local anaesthetic is needed. Anti-D should be given to all Rh negative women after the procedure.

DISEASES IN PREGNANCY

Asymptomatic bacteriuria

This affects about 5% of pregnant women. It may result in pyelonephritis in one-third of patients and there is some structural abnormality in 3–5%. All pregnant women should have their urine tested for the presence of white cells or culture for bacteria. Treatment depends on the organism isolated and the sensitivity.

Chronic renal disease

Most women with this condition are diagnosed before pregnancy.

The combination of leg oedema and proteinuria should suggest some renal involvement. All women with proteinuric hypertension should have their blood pressure and renal function checked on a regular basis, even after delivery.

The fetal prognosis depends on the gestation stage of the disease and the severity.

In recent years many pregnancies have been reported following renal transplantation. There is no evidence that pregnancy increased the incidence of renal rejection but proteinuric hypertension is twice as common in pregnancy following renal transplantation.

There is little evidence that immunosuppressant drugs or steroids are associated with an increased risk of congenital abnormalities.

Anaemia in pregnancy

The condition may follow blood loss, increased breakdown of red blood cells or lack of production of blood cells.

In pregnancy most anaemia is haemopoietic when it can be due to lack of iron, which causes iron deficiency anaemia, or folic acid, when a megaloblastic anaemia results. Iron deficiency anaemia in pregnancy may be the result of poor intake, poor absorption or increased utilization. It is commoner in women with multiple pregnancies or when the woman is parous.

The diagnosis is clinically supported by laboratory findings and treatment is best with prevention: iron should be given depending on the degree of anaemia and the stage of pregnancy.

Patient compliance is poor with regard to iron, especially as side effects are likely. Total dose iron infusion (rarely used nowadays) or even transfusion may be considered in some patients depending on the severity of the condition. However, the use of such procedures should be discouraged.

Folic acid deficiency anaemia

The diagnosis is suspected clinically when the pregnant woman is tired, breathless, with some oedema and possibly other signs of malnutrition. Folic acid supplement is not only beneficial in preventing anaemia, it is also beneficial in preventing neural tube defects.

In mild or moderate cases of folic acid deficiency anaemia folic acid 5–10 mg per day is therapeutic. In severe cases folic acid 5–10 mg per day is necessary; 5–10 mg per day intramuscularly may be given in such circumstances.

Heart problems in pregnancy

Rheumatic heart disease accounts for 80% of such cases, mostly mitral valve problems; 10% are usually due to aortic valve disease and 5% are a combination of mitral and aortic valve disease. Congenital heart disease accounts for 15% of the total.

Pregnancy may be tolerated with acyanotic congenital heart defects, but be aware of women with severe aortic stenosis and coarctation of the aorta.

With mitral stenosis there is usually pulmonary oedema, especially if the valve is tight and the heart is small. This is of course the commonest and often occurs in late pregnancy or immediately post-partum.

Right-sided congestive heart failure rarely settles in pregnancy, especially in women with pre-existing congestive heart failure.

In aortic stenosis, there is usually left-sided congestive failure.

In Eisenmenger's syndrome, with either right to left shunt or bidirectional shunt, there is usually a high risk of developing pulmonary hypertension.

Make sure that your patient attends for her antenatal care. Joint management with a consultant cardiologist is essential.

Coarctation of the aorta is another condition that must be considered in the reproductive age group. Following successful treatment there is no increased risk in pregnancy but there is a risk of rupture of a repair in late pregnancy and during labour.

Management of heart disease in pregnancy   Management includes early diagnosis by history, examination and proper assessment of the severity.

All women with heart problems should be referred to hospital, and should preferably be seen in joint clinics with the physician. An echocardiogram must be considered. A chest X-ray may be informative if performed before pregnancy (check medical notes).

Treatment depends upon the age, severity of the lesion, stage of pregnancy and functional decompensation.

These women should be followed thoroughly in hospital and advice for rest should be given.

In labour it is important to reduce the extra work by giving good analgesia, probably epidural, unless contraindicated.

Women in labour should be nursed head up, tilting the bed or the pillows. Antibiotic cover must be given, and obviate the need for excessive bearing down.

The use of forceps or vacuum extraction should shorten the second stage of labour. Syntometrine should be given if there is a high risk of developing post-partum haemorrhage and every effort should be made to prevent and treat pulmonary oedema if it develops.

Post-natal care is essential. These women should be followed-up thoroughly; they must have adequate rest and should be kept in hospital for a slightly longer time. Check home conditions prior to discharge.

Physiotherapy for the legs and gentle exercise are recommended and breastfeeding is not contraindicated unless the cardiac condition deteriorates in pregnancy.

The prognosis depends on the stage and the severity of the disease. Some women, for example those with metallic cardiac valves, require anti-coagulation during pregnancy. Referral to a specialist who deals with high-risk pregnant women is mandatory.

Respiratory disease in pregnancy

Asthma may worsen in pregnancy for emotional reasons, and asthma treatment should be continued throughout pregnancy.

Pregnancy is known to improve asthma in some patients, but in the puerperium it may recur with variable severity.

During labour, facial oxygen is useful. Delivery will improve respiratory effort. If the woman is on steroids the dosage should be adjusted during labour.

It is noted that the growth of babies may be affected due to poor control of asthma.

Pulmonary tuberculosis

This disease is becoming very rare in developed countries but is still high among migrants; recent reports suggest that there is an increase of the disease in the UK. History and examination usually point to a diagnosis: a patient with cough, dyspnoea or haemoptysis should be suspected of suffering from TB.

Management starts with notifying new cases to the district community physician; continue all anti-tuberculous drugs if these have been started, but be aware that there is a potentially teratogenic effect of some of these medications.

Bed-rest and family follow-up are essential. Delivery may be urgently required.

In the puerperium, breastfeeding may be allowed if the sputum for bacteriology is negative within 1 year with no active new lesion. All medication should be continued in the puerperium. If the baby has to be separated from the mother, suppression of lactation is indicated. A *multi-disciplinary* approach is indicated.

It is essential to consider the baby and whether or not the infant should be separated from the mother, especially if the sputum is still positive, but every effort must be taken to explain the reasons for this to the mother and her partner.

Endocrine disease in pregnancy

Thyroid problems in pregnancy. Oestrogen itself causes some enlargement of the thyroid gland and an increase in the output of thyroid hormones, but the clinical picture is of euthyroid.

Hypothyroidism is very rarely encountered in pregnancy, as such women are usually infertile. The condition of hyperthyroidism is very difficult to diagnose for the first time in pregnancy. If it was established before, treatment should continue in the form of carbimazole, and the dose could be increased. A physician's advice is essential.

Thyroidectomy, if considered because of poor control of the disease, could be performed in pregnancy, usually after the second trimester.

Radioactive iodine should be avoided in pregnancy.

Beware of neonatal thyrotoxicosis.

Pituitary diseases in pregnancy

Prolactinoma. Women who are on long-term medication for prolactinaemia could get pregnant while on these medications.

Oestrogen stimulation during pregnancy may cause an enlargement of the pituitary gland and the patient's vision may be threatened because of pressure.

A CT scan is essential for the diagnosis; prolactin level is not very accurate and of poor predictive value.

Rubella

This is becoming rare nowadays due to widespread vaccination; in the UK all pregnant women are routinely tested for the presence of rubella at booking.

If the woman is seronegative she should be vaccinated in the puerperium. Rubella infection rapidly crosses the placental barrier and may cause abnormalities in the fetus including congenital heart disease, deafness, mental retardation, microcephaly, hepatosplenomegaly and thrombocytopoenia if the mother is infected in the latter half of the pregnancy.

In early pregnancy, if a woman is suspected of having the disease, she should have a rubella-specific IgM test. If this is positive, management should be discussed thoroughly with the patient. If she considers termination of her pregnancy, this is justified if the primary infection was less that 10 weeks' gestation, as 50% of babies will be affected. Chorionic villus sampling may be indicated to detect whether or not the virus has crossed the placenta. The results are usually available within a short period of time enabling a valid decision.

A fetal blood sample between 18–20 weeks is indicated to determine if the IgM test is positive for rubella.

If negative the patient can be reassured, but if it is positive this confirms that the fetus has the infection although it does not indicate the presence of morphological abnormalites. Most women will, however, ask for termination of pregnancy once they have been informed about the results.

Cytomegalovirus (CMV)

This is the commonest perinatal infection in the UK. Manifestations include hepatosplenomegaly, jaundice, thromocytopoenia, chorioretinitis and infection that may result in stillbirth. The infant may be free of clinical manifestations until the *late* development of neurological disorders.

The disease may be acquired in an adult by sexual contact or blood transfusion, in the perinatal period by crossing the placenta, and also in childhood from other children's saliva, urine, stool or tears.

At present there is no vaccination for the disease. Careful counselling is important.

Toxoplasmosis

This is caused by the protozoan *Toxoplasma gondii*. The infection is usually acquired from cats, and human infection results from eating poorly cooked meals that contain the tissue cysts or food that was exposed to infected cat faeces.

The infection usually crosses the placenta and it may be asymptomatic in the mother but can in some cases produce a flu-like illness. It may result in cerebral calcifications, which may subsequently result in a space-occupying lesion, epilepsy or cerebral damage. It can also cause chorioamnionitis, hydrocephaly or microcephaly. The mother can usually be treated by antibiotics (spiramycin) that will prevent further transplacental damage. Fetal blood sampling is required to diagnose the disease in the fetus.

Human parvovirus B19

Another name for this disease is face disease or slapped-cheek syndrome; it is usually preceded by a non-specific febrile illness.

The infant is usually normal but the inhibition of fetal erythropoiesis can result which can cause fetal anaemia, hydrops and ascites.

In some centres treatment is possible by intrauterine transfusion to correct the abnormalities.

Herpes simplex virus (HSV)

Diagnosis is by culture in a special viral medium. Aciclovir cream reduces the duration of signs and symptoms.

In primary infection the risk of disease transmission from mother to fetus at vaginal delivery is high but very low if the infection is a recurrent type.

In primary infection with active genital lesions, delivery by Caesarean section should be considered if labour occurs and the membranes are intact, or within 4 hours of rupture of the membranes. Viral swabs from the baby are essential and treatment with aciclovir is indicated if the swabs are positive.

If the time between rupture of membranes and delivery is more than 4 hours, vaginal delivery should be allowed because Caesarean section is very unlikely to reduce the risk of neonatal infection.

Again, viral swabs are indicated and treatment with aciclovir is essential.

In secondary infection with active genital lesions the actual extent of the disease is not certain and treatment should follow the primary infection strategy.

A paediatrician should be informed of a suspected HSV infection in the neonate.

Hepatitis B virus

While most of people recover fully from this disease it is estimated that between 8–12% of the population become carriers after infection. There are significant geographical variations in the prevalence of HBV infection. Screening is essential at booking.

There is a significant risk to the fetus if the mother has had a recent infection or if she is a carrier with antibodies to the E antigen. Infants of HBsAG-positive mothers should be given hepatitis B gammaglobulin within 12 hours after birth and an initial dose of hepatitis B vaccine within 7 days.

Another dose of vaccine at 1 and 6 months should be given and testing for antibodies should be perfomed at 12 and 15 months. A paediatrician should be involved.

Hepatitis C virus

This is the major cause of the non-A, non-B post-transfusion hepatitis; many sporadic hepatitis cases in western Europe and the USA result from this disease. Up to 80% of the infected population will become chronic carriers.

Vertical transmission through the placenta is minimal. No routine screening is, therefore, necessary for the time being.

Human immunodeficiency virus (HIV)

Drug abuse is the main method of transmission in the UK although unprotected heterosexual intercourse carries an accepted level of risk. HIV is epidemic in Africa and it is reported that up to 30% of pregnant women are infected. The risk from vertical transmission varies and different percentages have been given but it could be between 10–30%.

Transmission itself depends on many factors such as virus load and the presence or absence of neutralizing antibody, together with the mode of delivery and whether or not the woman is going to breastfeed her child.

Antenatal testing is practised in certain high-risk areas. Involvement of a physician with an interest in HIV is essential in the management of these patients, as well as a paediatrician. Infection control policies should be strictly adhered to.

Care in labour and the post-natal period should be carried out by experienced professionals.

In labour it is important to avoid fetal scalp clips and fetal blood sampling to minimize the risk of transmission.

Mouth-operated suction devices should be avoided with such patients.

Streptococcal infection

This may cause pre-term rupture of the membranes and consequently pre-term labour. In certain instances severe post-partum infection occurs, especially following Caesarean section, and overwhelming neonatal infection may lead to death. One in five women will carry group B streptococci in the vagina and 1/50 will give birth to an infected infant; about 1/5000 women will lose an infant due to overwhelming sepsis.

Screening of all pregnant women for infection is not practised at the moment but it should be offered to 'at risk' groups of the population.

Listeriosis

About 3% of pregnant women carry listeria organisms in the rectum. It may also be acquired in pregnancy from eating unpasteurized cheese and from uncooked meats.

Infection may result in maternal diarrhoea accompanied by a temperature, meconium staining of the amniotic fluid in a very pre-term baby and/or premature labour. Treatment is by intravenous ampicillin.

Syphilis

Screening for this disease, despite the fact that it is not common, is still cost effective. The primary lesion appears as a chancre at the site of inoculation.

Secondary syphilis usually occurs between 6–12 weeks after the initial lesion and it consists of a skin rash, low-grade temperature, general illness and generalized lymphadenopathy. Hepatomegaly may occur.

If not treated early, infection may result in premature delivery or perinatal death.

Congenital syphilis results in lasting neurological and skeletal damage. Management includes the use of penicillin and involvement of a paediatrician and genitourinary physician. Contact tracing is essential and the disease is notifiable.

Diabetes mellitus

This condition is diagnosed when the fasting glucose venous plasma concentration is equal to or exceeds 8 mmol/l or if the venous glucose plasma concentration equals or exceeds 11.0 mmol/l 2 h after a 75 g oral glucose load.

Symptoms of diabetes include polydipsia, weight loss despite good appetite and polyuria. During antenatal booking the primary cause of diabetes mellitus should be suspected in a woman with persistent glycosuria on two occasions antenatally or a single fasting urine sample. Always note the time food was taken before the testing.

Other risk factors include a woman with a family history of diabetes, previous big babies, diabetes in a previous pregnancy, unexpected stillbirth or neonatal death, maternal obesity and polyhydramnios.

Antenatal screening is essential as about 30% of women with gestational diabetes have none of the above risk factors and not all women with impaired glucose tolerance or even frank diabetes have persistent glycosuria, and glycosuria may sometimes occur once or twice during a normal pregnancy.

Poorly controlled diabetes may result in retinopathy, nephropathy and neuropathy which may deteriorate without treatment. There is also an increased risk of congenital malformation which is related to hyperglycaemia during organogenesis. Sacral agenesis is rare but characteristically associated with poor diabetic control.

Obstetric complications in the form of polyhydramnios, pre-term labour and pre-eclampsia are commoner with poor control. Urinary and genital infections are also known to occur.

The incidence of sudden unexpected fetal death increases with poor control of diabetes. Shoulder dystocia and neonatal problems which range from birth trauma, hyaline membrane disease, hypoglycaemia, hypocalcaemia, hypomagnesaemia and/or jaundice are all known associations with poor control of diabetes.

Ideally management should start with a pre-pregnancy counselling clinic outlining plans for the pregnancy including dietary advice, infection screening, blood glucose monitoring and routine screening procedures.

The GP plays an important role in highlighting these issues. It is important to identify young diabetic women and document how long they have been diabetic. A known diabetic woman should be treated jointly by an obstetrician and a dietician to establish optimal diabetic control. The dietician should advise the correct calorie intake and carbohydrate content.

A blood glucose profile should be performed twice a week and the urine analysed on a regular basis.

Glycosylated haemoglobin provides retrospective information on the validity of glucose monitoring. When necessary, soluble and intermediate acting insulin types should be used in the morning and evening.

Intermittent soluble insulin should be used with each meal and intermediate-acting insulin in the evening.

Human or highly profiled porcine insulin reduces the risk of developing antibodies.

Management of diabetes in pregnancy requires monitoring of both mother and the fetus.

Regular check-ups of the mother, especially assessing blood pressure and renal function, with regular examination of the fundi, are all important in monitoring the condition.

Baseline fetal assessment to confirm gestational age and a detailed scan at 18–20 weeks to exclude morphological abnormalities, especially cranial, spinal and cardiac defects, are mandatory. Serial growth monitoring is essential and regular assessment of fetal wellbeing is necessary in the third trimester.

Gestational diabetes

This is a condition occurring during pregnancy in which the serum glucose returns to normal following pregnancy.

Initially management may be by dietary control but if this fails insulin could be given. Delivery is usually by induction of labour at term provided that fetal and maternal conditions are acceptable.

During labour close control of blood glucose is achieved by continuous infusion of soluble insulin and a separate infusion of 5% dextrose with added potassium chloride (KCl). Regular blood pressure and close monitoring should be undertaken and the intravenous fusion titrated to keep levels between 5–7 mmol/l.

Appropriate fetal monitoring is also required.

Epilepsy in pregnancy

Pre-conception counselling is of great importance in women who suffer from epilepsy in order to review their drug therapy and seizure control.

It should be stressed that pregnancy does not provoke epilepsy, but the frequency of seizures may increase as a result of rapid clearance of anti-convulsant therapy. The risk of an epileptic mother having an epileptic child is about 1 in 44.

Drugs are not without risk in pregnancy and it is important to note that cleft lip and/or palate, congenital heart defects, possible characteristic facial appearances and retarded growth are all known effects of medication used for epilepsy. It is, however, important to prescribe anti-convulsants in doses sufficient to prevent convulsions. This should be done in close liaison with the specialist physician. It is always advisable to aim for one treatment if possible.

Vitamin K should be given to all neonates and breastfeeding should be encouraged. Should status epilepticus occur intravenous diazepam is important and the airway must be kept patent. Oxygen is usually given.

A proper explanation to the mother after her seizure is important and further counselling is indicated.

Jaundice in pregnancy

The incidence is usually 1–2 per 1500 pregnancies; intrahepatic cholestasis accounts for about one-fifth of the cases.

The patient usually presents with pruritus in the second half of pregnancy. There is an elevated serum bilirubin and transaminase. There is a known association with pre-term delivery, *fetal compromise and stillbirth*. Jaundice usually eases off after delivery and no chronic liver damage is expected.

Recurrence of the condition is likely and it may also occur in association with the contraceptive pill. Colestyramine will reduce itching but is very unpleasant to take. If the jaundice is prolonged vitamin K should be given.

Intercurrent jaundice in pregnancy Causes of this include viral hepatitis, cholelithiasis, drug toxicity and haemolysis. The viral hepatitis is usually due to hepatitis B or C and this accounts for 40% of cases. Cholelithiasis accounts for 5%.

The diagnosis may be confirmed by ultrasound and cholecystectomy may be carried out in pregnancy if necessary.

Drug toxicity and haemolysis are very rare causes of jaundice but always check the information sheets of medication given to women in pregnancy.

Other problems in pregnancy

Coeliac disease. This may present as a folate deficiency anaemia. If not treated there is an increased risk of miscarriage and intrauterine growth retardation. A gluten-free diet and vitamins are important methods of management.

Ulcerative colitis. There is no adverse effect on the condition in pregnancy and the pregnancy does not increase the chance of relapse of ulcerative colitis but if the colitis arises in pregnancy or during the puerperium the prognosis is usually worse. Rectal steroids and sulfasalazines are given during pregnancy.

Crohn's disease. There is a slightly increased adverse effect in the fetal outcome with Crohn's disease in pregnancy but the condition is not affected by pregnancy. There may be a deterioration during the puerperium.

Treatment is no different from in the non-pregnant stage.

Thromboembolism and thrombosis

Thrombosis, thromboembolism and hypertensive disease of pregnancy are the major causes of maternal death in the UK. The exact figures of maternal deaths may be found in Confidential Enquiries into Maternal Deaths.

There is a slight increase in the risk of thrombosis in cases of elective Caesarean section in an otherwise uncomplicated pregnancy and for women in this group with a slight risk, early mobilization and hydration are mandatory.

Moderate risk includes women over the age of 35, parity of four or more, increased body mass index, gross varicose veins, emergency Caesarean section, sickle-cell disease and pre-eclampsia. For the mother in the 'at risk' group prophylaxis should be considered.

The 'high risk' group includes those conditions named as moderate risk but to a greater degree, as well as a positive family history of thrombosis, thrombophilia, anti-cardiolipin syndrome, the presence of lupus inhibitor or a major operation such as Caesarean hysterectomy. In this high-risk group heparin and leg stockings should be used.

Deep-vein thrombosis (DVT) complicates about 1–2% of severe infections. Diagnosis is suspected clinically when the woman complains of pain, local tenderness, swelling and oedema. Homan's sign is not reliable.

Be aware of the silent deep-vein thrombosis and do not rely on clinical signs and symptoms in diagnosing the disease.

The majority of cases of DVT occur on the left side. Venography and Doppler scan are also used in diagnosis of the condition.

Pulmonary embolus

The condition may arise with clinical evidence of DVT. It gives severe pleuritic pain which may be associated with dyspnoea and haemoptysis. Shock may occur in varying degrees. Pyrexia, bronchospasm and tachycardia are associated developments of the pulmonary embolism.

Chest X-ray, although indicated, may be completely normal as may ECG, except when the embolus is of massive size and has already produced acute cor pulmonale.

A VQ lung scan is essential (ventilation perfusion isotope) and in some cases angiography may be indicated.

Treatment of deep-vein thrombosis and pulmonary embolus is an emergency which should be dealt with immediately. Treatment is with heparin, which inhibits thrombin, and factors VIII, X, XI, XII.

In acute cases intravenous heparin, 40 000 units daily for at least 48 hours, should be considered and long-term therapy with subcutaneous heparin is essential to inhibit activated factor X without prolonging the clotting time. Twice daily therapy of this or low molecular heparin is of great value.

Remember that the use of heparin does not act as a risk of haemorrhage even when an operative delivery is indicated.

Therapy should continue for 6 weeks after the acute attack.

Warfarin is to be avoided in the first trimester of pregnancy because of the slight risk of teratogenesis. Fetal haemorrhage may also arise because of the use of warfarin. The difference between heparin and warfarin is that the effect of warfarin cannot be reversed quickly, and warfarin should be continued for at least 6 weeks after delivery.

Dextran 70 has been used in the past but is best avoided in pregnancy. It is essential to involve the haematologist in the management of all thrombotic diseases.

Autoimmune thrombocytopenia (ITP)
There is fetal risk from this condition, the main problem being intracranial haemorrhage.
Caesarean section does not reduce the risk of intracranial haemorrhage.
The mother should be investigated thoroughly and treatment should involve the haematologist and the specialist physician in autoimmune disease. Corticosteroids, platelet transfusion and plasmapheresis are the lines of treatment.

Systemic lupus erythematosus (SLE)
This is a multi-system disorder of unknown origin and it can affect women in the reproductive age group. The diagnosis depends on the presence of certain criteria and pregnancy has no specific effects on SLE, although the condition may worsen during the puerperium.
It is known that women with SLE may suffer miscarriages, hypertension in pregnancy and lupus nephritis.
Management should include the haematologist and a specialist physician.

Rhesus ISO-immunization
Sensitization may occur during the antenatal period in up to 2% of previously unsensitized or Rh negative women.
It usually arises due to fetal/maternal haemorrhage during labour or miscarriage. Prevention is by giving anti-D in defined doses dependent on the gestation. It is important for the GP to check whether anti-D was given when indicated. Early referral to hospital once the antibodies are detected is mandatory and treatment will depend on the severity of the condition.

LABOUR

Normal labour is characterized by uterine contractions causing dilatation of the cervix and descent of the presenting part.
There are three stages of labour and progress is usually assessed with the partogram which provides a visual record of the labour including cervical dilatation, descent of the presenting part, contractions, fetal heart rate, liquor, the time when the membranes ruptured, moulding of the fetal skull, oxytocin used and vital signs of the mother.
Normal labour is usually managed by midwifery staff.

Induction of labour
The artificial rupture of membranes (with subsequent commencement of labour) is a method of inducing labour if it is acceptable to mother. The patient's requests should be respected, and each case decided upon its merits.
Contraindications for inducing labour include abnormal lie, two or more previous Caesarean sections for recurrent reasons such as cephalopelvic disproportion, and if there is a fibroid or a tumour occupying the pelvis.

It is essential to check on the gestational age before embarking on any induction. Induction can be scheduled for cervical ripening using prostaglandin.

After artificial rupture of the membranes an oxytocin infusion may also be the method of use in inducing labour. Augmentation is another term for acceleration of labour.

Pre-term labour and delivery

By definition this is labour occurring before 37 completed weeks. It accounts for 3–10% of all deliveries and is a major cause of neonatal death. Pre-term labour may have no known cause, the majority being maternal or fetal conditions other than multiple pregnancy in about 25% of cases.

Multiple pregnancy itself accounts for 10% of cases of prematurity, while iatrogenic factors account for 25% of instances of pre-term labour.

Certain conditions are associated with pre-term labour including antepartum haemorrhage, intrauterine growth retardation, cervical incompetence, diabetes, polyhydramnios, renal problems, congenitally defined abnormalities, multiple pregnancy and intrauterine infections.

It is very difficult to predict pre-term labour, but at risk groups should be checked thoroughly and regularly in hospital.

Corticosteroid therapy given to mothers between 24–34 weeks has made a significant improvement in fetal lung maturity.

Beta-sympathomimetic drugs to inhibit labour should be given cautiously, and there are contraindications for this medication especially antepartum haemorrhage, pre-eclampsia, maternal heart problems and thyrotoxicosis.

The medication should be considered in cases when steroids are given time to work or when a transfer is to be arranged to a tertiary referral centre.

Management of women who present with premature rupture of the membranes

This depends on the time that has elapsed since the membranes ruptured. Generally speaking conservative management should be considered before inducing labour. The majority of these will go into spontaneous labour at 24–48 h. Delivery may be indicated if there are risks to the mother or to the fetus.

Management of normal labour

Stages of labour   The first stage of labour is defined as lasting from the onset of labour until the cervix is fully dilated. The second stage is from full cervical dilatation to the complete expulsion of the baby. The third stage lasts from the time when the fetus is expelled until expulsion of the placenta and accompanying membranes.

Management of normal labour starts with a diagnosis of labour. A midwife or a general practitioner should advise the pregnant woman to attend hospital when the uterine contractions are occurring very regularly and painfully and/or when there is a rupture of the membranes.

Partograms are usually used to monitor the progress of labour.

Pain relief in labour   This topic is best discussed with an anaesthetist, and the mother should have her choices explained to her. The methods of pain relief include inhalation agents such as nitrous oxide, a TENS machine (transcutaneous electrical nerve stimulation), and narcotic medications such as pethidine, morphine and meptazinol.

There are also varieties of non-drug analgesia including hypnosis, transcutaneous nerve stimulation and acupuncture.

Epidural analgesia is widely used, and some units provide the service on a 24-hour basis.

There are certain complications associated with epidural analgesia, however, and these include a dural tap, total spinal block or hypotension. There is also the risk of prolongation of the second stage which may require an instrumental delivery.

Anaesthesia may be required for operative delivery. Regional anaesthesia in the form of a spinal and epidural block are commonly used, although general anaesthesia is used in some cases.

Monitoring during labour   This depends on the gestational age and whether the pregnancy is labelled as high, moderate or low risk.

Low-risk pregnancies are intermittently monitored but continuous fetal monitoring is advised for the high-risk group which includes pre-term infants, intrauterine growth retardation, multiple pregnancies, breech presentation or where the mother has a medical condition. Most units in the UK use continuous fetal monitoring with CTG and fetal blood sampling if indicated.

Passage of meconium in labour   If the pregnancy is not post mature or the presenting part is breech the passage of meconium may indicate fetal compromise and therefore prompt delivery in some cases.

Management of abnormal labour   Abnormal labour may present in the first or second stage, and careful assessment is essential to identify the possible cause.

Cephalopelvic disproportion   This diagnosis is rare in Caucasians but commoner in Africans and Afro-Caribbeans. The various methods of assessing cephalopelvic disproportion are not accurate and the best pelvimetry is the passage of the presenting part in labour; this is why trial of labour is justified in almost all cases.

Mapresentations and malposition   Breech presentation occurs in 2–3% of all labours, posing a problem when this presents as undiagnosed breech in labour. Breech presentation may arise from various causes.

Congenital abnormalities should be considered as well as other conditions that affect the lower segment.

There are three types of breech presentation: flexed, extended and the footling type. Fully flexed means that both legs are flexed at the hip and knee; it is also referred to as complete or flexed breech.

An extended breech occurs when neither knee joints flex, so that both legs are extended; it is also called frank breech or breech with extended legs, and this type is the commonest presentation.

Sometimes the breech may present with one leg flexed and the other leg extended: hence the term footling or incomplete breech. A footling breech occurs commonly with very tiny babies and in pre-term pregnancies.

The diagnosis of breech is made very easy by the use of an ultrasound scan, although vaginal examination is sometimes necessary to confirm the presenting part.

Management of breech depends on many factors. There are certain criteria required allowing vaginal breech delivery, including ultrasound scan to determine the type of breech, estimated fetal weight and exclusion of congenital abnormalities and placenta praevia.

Management of breech in labour depends on the progress, so careful assessment of progress is essential. Syntocinon may be given in the first stage in some cases.

If Syntocinon was not used earlier, it should *not* be used in the second stage. Any abnormalities in either the first or second stage necessitate an urgent Caesarean section.

The patient and her partner should be counselled thoroughly concerning all anticipated problems relating to breech delivery.

External cephalic version   ECV is encouraged as a method of changing the presenting part and this should be done with the patient's agreement after 36 weeks' gestation.

The patient should be counselled regarding the risks, which are as follows: it may stimulate labour, spontaneous rupture of membranes, abruption or – on rare occasions – intrauterine fetal death. Rh-negative women should receive anti-D. Careful monitoring is essential as the procedure is performed.

Transverse lie   This occurs in less than 1% of all deliveries. It may be due to polyhydramnios or when the head or the presenting part is prevented from going into the pelvis, for reasons such as a fibroid, cephalopelvic disproportion or placenta praevia.

Transverse lie may present as a result of uterine abnormalities and it is common in the second twin. Multiparity is another common cause of transverse or unstable lie. Caesarean section is indicated. Even this method of delivery should be performed by an experienced obstetrician because of anticipated problems with transverse lie.

Face presentation This occurs in 1% of all deliveries. The many reasons for it include deflexed fetal head or lax uterus. It is common in multiparous mothers and in women with polyhydramnios. The diagnosis is usually established during labour and an experienced obstetrician should decide the mode of delivery and preferably conduct labour.

Occipito-posterior position This is the commonest problem facing many obstetricians and midwives, and the incidence depends on the population.

Diagnosis can be made antenatally during the routine assessment visit. In labour, the occipito-posterior position may be identified on vaginal examination.

During labour most of the cases will progress normally and deliver spontaneously, but in some cases assisted delivery will be necessary.

Brow presentation Again this occurs in less than 1% of all deliveries. The diagnosis is usually apparent during labour and management of it requires an experienced obstetrician to decide the mode of delivery, which is usually by Caesarean section.

Cord prolapse and cord presentation During labour, loops of the umbilical cord may be felt ahead of the presenting part. If the membranes are intact the condition is termed cord presentation and is not dangerous but delivery should still be imminent.

If the cord prolapse occurs with ruptured membranes and a live baby, this necessitates urgent delivery.

If the cervix is not dilated enough emergency Caesarean section should be performed.

Post-partum haemorrhage (PPH)

Post-partum haemorrhage is defined in different ways but usually as bleeding from the genital tract after delivery of the fetus.

It is defined as primary when the blood loss is in excess of 500 ml within 24 hours of birth. Secondary PPH occurs after the completed 24 hours. It is caused by genital tract trauma, retained products of conception and/or uterine atony.

The diagnosis is usually obvious and treatment should be prompt, as this is a known cause of maternal death. Oxytocin should be given with delivery of the baby: Syntometrine, for example, is routinely given as an i.m. injection after the delivery of the anterior shoulder in most units and this reduces the incidence of death.

If PPH occurs another dose of oxytocin should be given; blood should be crossmatched and the cause of the PPH should be identified and treated accordingly.

Secondary PPH is defined as abnormal vaginal bleeding that occurs after the first 24 hours. The woman usually presents with the passage of clots after 7–10 days with resumption of fresh vaginal bleeding. This may be due to retained products of conception, either the placenta or membranes, or the residual decidua may become necrotic and infected.

All such patients should be referred to hospital for admission and appropriate treatment should be provided.

Multiple pregnancy in labour

With twins pre-term labour is common. Placenta praevia may be present, and malpresentations are frequently observed.

The usual presentation is vertex vertex but combinations include: vertex breech, breech vertex, breech breech, vertex transverse and breech transverse. In cases of breech breech, Caesarean section is indicated.

Management of labour and delivery should be conducted by a multi-disciplinary team. An intravenous line should be set up and an anaesthetist and a paediatrician should be informed.

After the delivery of the first twin, the lie of the second twin should be assessed. If the lie is longitudinal the second sac should be ruptured once uterine activity begins. Any delay of more than 20 minutes after the delivery of the first twin necessitates an urgent delivery.

Operative deliveries

Episiotomy is the most common procedure performed in obstetric units. It may be indicated when a perineal tear appears inevitable or in cases of fetal distress late in the second stage. Episiotomy should be performed at the correct time and carried out with adequate anaesthesia.

Third degree tear   This results when the vaginal laceration or episiotomy has extended to involve at least the anal mucosa, and must be repaired in theatre under epidural, spinal or general anaesthesia. A low residual diet and faecal softening agent should be given for about 5–7 days. The woman should be counselled regarding the tear and reassured.

Instrumental delivery   This includes ventouse and forceps deliveries, and prerequisites for an instrumental delivery are: a valid indication must be present and the presentation must be suitable, for example a vertex or a face, or sometimes the aftercoming head in breech delivery. Cephalopelvic disproportion should be ruled out. The presenting part must be engaged and the membranes ruptured.

Abdominally, the head should not be palpable and if more than one-fifth can be palpated vaginal delivery should be abandoned.

The position of the fetal head must be known and the cervix fully dilated; and the bladder should preferably be emptied by catheterisation.

Adequate analgesia should be used and the uterus must be contracting. Instrumental deliveries are learnt in the labour ward and no instrumental delivery should be performed if there is any question of its safety.

Caesarean section   There has been an increase in the number of Caesarean section deliveries in recent years. The matter is complicated by the patient's demands.

There are two types of indication for Caesarean section: maternal indication or fetal indication.

Most Caesarean sections are performed under an epidural and the woman should be counselled regarding the delivery. The partner usually attends if no complication is expected.

THE PUERPERIUM

The puerperium is the time when the mother is returning to her pre-pregnant state, and this it usually takes about 6 weeks. There are many physiological changes in the genital tract during this time.

The community midwife and the GP should be aware of these changes. In the first week, temperature, lochia, blood pressure, uterine size, urine output and bowel habit should be assessed. The serum Hb should be measured on day 4 if the blood loss exceeds the expected level. Exercise is encouraged and diet should be adequate. Feeding should be discussed and the mother should be supported with the method she chooses.

Psychological support is essential for a woman in the puerperium and regular post-natal visits should be arranged with the community midwives. Contraception should be discussed when the time is right.

Psychiatric problems in the puerperium

The baby blues   Some women feel depressed on the 3rd to 5th day after delivery. This is usually a short-lived problem but the clinician should look for complications such as anaemia, inadequate sleep, delayed healing from an episiotomy or Caesarean section, or a delay in establishing breastfeeding. Post-partum pyrexia is a known cause of extended baby blues.

Treatment is supportive. Some women may present with depression and here a psychiatrist should be involved early in the management.

Post-partum psychosis   This is extremely rare and occurs in 1 woman per 1000, but it can be life threatening for mother or baby.

It presents with delusion and confusion, and in some cases rejection of the newborn. Management should be admission to the mother and baby unit and appropriate psychotherapeutic medications should be given.

Post-partum pyrexia   This is a temperature at or over 38°C on two occasions more than 4 hours apart. It may be related to an infection of the urinary tract, chest, breast or genital tract, and may sometimes may be due to thromboembolic episodes.

The organisms which are usually identified vary but *Streptococcus faecalis*, staphylococcus group E, haemolytic streptococcus or *E. coli* are commonly detected in blood cultures and vaginal swabs.

The history usually suggests the diagnosis and investigations should be performed, especially a white blood cell count and high vaginal swab. Management is admission and an appropriate antibiotic regimen. Look for a urinary tract infection or breast abscess as a source of the post-partum pyrexia.

Pulmonary embolism (see p. 204).

NOTES ON NEONATAL PAEDIATRICS 7

COMMON NEONATAL PROBLEMS

Jaundice

This is a common problem in neonates, with around 50% of babies becoming jaundiced in the first few days of life. It may be of physiological origin, caused by immature liver enzymes, a high haemoglobin load and increased enterohepatic circulation. The serum bilirubin peaks around day 3 and then fades over the next few days. It also may be pathological; this should be suspected if it occurs in the first 24 hours, lasts more than 10 days, or is associated with illness.

Common causes are haemolysis (caused by Rhesus disease, ABO incompatibility, and glucose-6-phosphate dehydrogenase deficiency), and infections such as those of the urinary tract. Metabolic causes such as galactosaemia are rare but important.

Investigations should include serum bilirubin level, blood group and direct Coombs test (for haemolysis), haemoglobin and urine for culture and reducing substances. Bruising and polycythaemia also predispose a baby to jaundice.

Treatment may not be required, or may consist of phototherapy, combined with adequate fluid intake. If the serum bilirubin is very high (usually above 450 μmol/l in a term baby) then an exchange transfusion may be required to prevent kernicterus and irreversible neurological damage.

Prolonged jaundice is defined as hyperbilirubinaemia lasting greater than 10 days in a term baby, or greater than 14 days in a pre-term infant. It is commonly caused by breastfeeding, but this is a diagnosis of exclusion in a healthy baby. Investigations should be undertaken without delay, as the jaundice may be an indication of serious illness.

If conjugated, consider biliary atresia, neonatal hepatitis or cystic fibrosis. If unconjugated, consider hypothyroidism or infection.

Investigations should include urine for culture, thyroid function testing, liver function, and a total and conjugated bilirubin level.

Skin rashes

These are often a cause of worry for mothers at neonatal check-up.

Erythema toxicum occurs in half of all babies, usually in the first 48 hours of life. Its appearance may be erythematous patches or small pustules. It is benign, and parents should be reassured.

Milia are small pearly white papules over the nose. These resolve with time and are harmless.

'Stork marks' or salmon patches are naevi seen on the eyelids or between the brows, and on the nape of the neck. Most resolve, although a small number of the neck lesions persist, but will usually be covered by the hairline.

Port-wine stains are usually present at birth, but parents must *not* be told that these will resolve, as they do *not* disappear with time.

Erb's palsy

This condition is caused by brachial plexus injury, commonly seen in large babies after difficult deliveries. The arm is held pronated and internally rotated (waiter's tip position) after damage to C5 and C6 nerve roots.

Prognosis is generally good with a recovery rate of 75–95%; however early surgery is showing better outcomes for non-improvers. Babies should therefore have an early review appointment.

Congenital dislocation of the hip

Hip clicks are common and are usually insignificant, but if there is any doubt this can be resolved by ultrasound.

The incidence of congenital dislocation is 1–2%. Risk factors include female sex, breech delivery and a family history of dislocated hips.

Ortolani and Barlow screening tests are performed at the neonatal check, but this may leave some babies undiagnosed. Many units perform hip ultrasound scans on all at risk births.

Talipes

This refers to the turning or twisting of the foot so that it cannot be placed flat on a flat surface. It may be related to neuromuscular disease or oligohydramnios.

Most respond to physiotherapy, and few need correctional surgery.

Cephalhaematoma

This is a soft swelling seen on the head that is caused by a collection of blood between the skull bones and the periosteum. It does not cross suture lines.

It is benign in outcome, and resolves in around 6 weeks.

Undescended testes

These should be taken seriously at all times. Testes which are palpable in the inguinal canal may descend into the scrotum in the first 3 months, but never drop after the age of 1 year.

Any baby with an undescended testicle at neonatal check should be kept under regular review, and if the testicle has not descended by the age of 1 then referral to a paediatric surgeon is necessary as there is a risk of malignancy later in life in the undescended organ.

Bilateral undescended testes may be an indicator of a more major endocrine or chromosomal abnormality and the baby should be examined very carefully for associated features.

NUTRITION

Breast versus bottle feeding

Breastfeeding is encouraged in the UK, particularly for mothers of pre-term infants where expressed breast milk is given via a nasogastric tube. It has been shown to be better tolerated by these babies and to be protective of the gut. Breast feeding is also thought to lead to better intellectual development. It contains many agents that protect against infection.

Appropriate support is necessary for inexperienced mothers. Many hospitals have midwifery staff dedicated to the promotion of breastfeeding with a special interest in the subject. In addition to this lay breastfeeding counsellors are available for mothers in the community, often associated with the National Childbirth Trust or the La Leche League.

Most babies are able to breastfeed, including many with abnormalities such as cleft lip and palate or micrognathia.

Feeding difficulties

These are common on the post-natal wards, particularly in babies born before 37 weeks.

The problem may usually be managed without admission to the baby unit. It is important to consider whether the mother has enough milk, and that the baby is able to latch onto the breast.

The baby should be examined thoroughly to ensure there are no signs of illness such as infection or intestinal obstruction.

If a long period has elapsed between feeds then blood sugar should be checked; if this is normal then it is best to persist with feeding on the post-natal ward with the support of experienced nursing staff.

Vitamin K

There is much controversy attached to vitamin K administration. It is given to prevent haemorrhagic disease of the newborn, a potentially lethal bleeding disorder.

Traditionally, 1 mg was given intramuscularly in the delivery room; however, in 1992 a paper was published proposing a link between i.m. vitamin K and childhood cancers including lymphoma and leukaemia. Subsequent work, which has been extensive, has failed to confirm this link.

Nevertheless, many hospitals have now changed their administration policy, and each chooses their own regimen.

Commonly 1 mg of an oral preparation is given, which may be followed up by further doses in the community. These further doses may depend on whether or not the baby is bottle fed (formula feeds are fortified with vitamin K). Other units continue to give i.m. vitamin K, but sometimes in a smaller dose.

NEONATAL SCREENING

Neonatal check

This is carried out at around 24 hours of age depending on local policy. It is a screening check for congenital abnormalities which have not previously been noted.

The check is usually carried out by paediatric or obstetric SHOs. It consists of the head-to-toe examination of an undressed baby, beginning with examination of the face and head for dysmorphic features, auscultation of the heart, examination of the palate and viewing of the red reflex. Palpation of the abdomen is carried out with assessment of the genitalia, hip examination and a brief neurological assessment including fontanelles, tone and primitive reflexes.

The usefulness of this is controversial: a significant percentage of heart murmurs cannot be detected in the first few days of life. Some units perform two checks, with one at discharge.

Metabolic screening

This varies between regions in the UK, and usually consists of a heelprick blood test undertaken by the midwife in the second week of life, depending on local policy.

The blood is then transported either in containers or on blotting paper to the regional screening labs where it is tested for hypothyroidism and phenylketonuria. Some regions also test for other metabolic diseases as well as cystic fibrosis.

Child health surveillance

On discharge from hospital mother and baby are visited by a community midwife for 2–4 weeks. When this ceases a health visitor will take on supervision of the child, providing regular input and advice on feeding, sleeping, development and immunization.

A formal review takes place at 6–8 weeks, and is performed by the GP or community paediatrician. This consists of a screening examination in the same form as the neonatal check and includes a developmental check. The first immunization is often given at this visit.

Immunization

This is largely guided by national policy, with only minor local variations. BCG may be offered at birth in certain areas where risk is considered high, or babies may be selected according to risk or racial origin.

At 2, 3 and 4 months babies are offered immunization against *Haemophilus influenzae* type b (Hib), *diphtheria, tetanus, pertussis, polio* and *meningococcus* type c.

Measles, mumps and *rubella* (MMR) vaccination is offered at 12–15 months.

The schedule of immunization changes according to current need and should be reviewed at regular intervals.

PROBLEMS OF PREMATURITY

Outcome and viability

The following are useful statistics regarding prematurity.

- Outcome is still poor at early gestation.
- Recent work shows that at 23 weeks only 12% of babies survived to discharge and 5% were neurologically intact.
- At 24 weeks 26% survived to discharge, 12% intact.
- At 25 weeks 45% survived to discharge, with 23% neurologically intact.

Surfactant deficient lung disease

This is also known as respiratory distress syndrome, and is most common in premature babies although it is also found in 1% of term babies, particularly those with disposing factors such maternal diabetes. It is commoner in boys and in certain families.

It presents with tachypnoea, sternal recession, grunting and cyanosis, which begins before 4 hours of age and persists beyond 24 hours of age. It may be prevented, or its severity reduced, by the use of antenatal steroids.

The natural history of the condition consists of worsening for 48–72 hours, then a plateau, followed by recovery by 1 week of age.

Management is largely support of the baby, providing ventilatory support which may range from facial oxygen to full ventilation.

Surfactant therapy is now available, and is administered via the ET tube as early in the illness as possible. Two types exist: natural and synthetic. The former is more effective.

Chronic lung disease

This is, also known as bronchopulmonary dysplasia. The infant shows coarse reticular shadowing on chest X-ray and has a persistent oxygen requirement at 28 days of age, or at 36 weeks post-conception.

It is commoner in white males and is thought to have multi-factorial causes, including oxygen toxicity and barotrauma caused by artificial ventilation.

Prevention is felt to be the best form of management, using the lowest oxygen concentration possible and the most gentle forms of ventilation.

Retinopathy of prematurity
This is a disorder of the developing retinal vasculature, where overgrowth of new vessels occurs, the progression of which may lead to scarring, retinal detachment and blindness.

Most cases resolve spontaneously. There is multi-factorial causation related to oxygen therapy and immaturity.

Intraventricular haemorrhage
This is a major cause of mortality in pre-term infants, often with cerebral infarct, caused by surges in blood pressure through fragile cerebral vessels, usually in the first 72 hours of life.

Prevention is by minimal handling of the infant, adequate pain relief and maintenance of a stable blood pressure.

White matter damage
Found in some pre-term babies, this can also occur antenatally, intrapartum or post-natally. It is a significant cause of neurological morbidity.

GROWTH PROBLEMS

Normal growth
Normal term neonates will lose around 10% of their birth weight in the first few days of life. They should have regained this weight by 10 days of age.

Pre-term or sick neonates will lose a higher percentage and take longer to regain the weight.

Small for gestational age
This refers to all babies born below the 10th centile for weight. They are prone to numerous problems including hypoglycaemia, hypothermia, polycythaemia, hypoxic ischaemic encephalopathy and behavioural problems later in childhood. It is important therefore that all small for gestational age babies should be kept warm after birth, be given early and regular feeds and have their blood sugar checked on a regular basis.

CONGENITAL ABNORMALITIES

Diaphragmatic hernia
In this condition the bowel and other abdominal viscera herniate through the diaphragm into the thoracic cavity.

The commonest is Bochdalek's hernia, which occurs in the posterolateral position, 80% occurring on the left side. Most are diagnosed on antenatal ultrasound scan, and the baby is then electively delivered in a regional centre with neonatal surgical facilities. The main difficulty for these babies is that pulmonary hypoplasia may accompany the anomaly, making survival precarious. Surgery is performed electively when the baby is stable and this is usually followed by a period of ventilatory support. Around 50% of babies with Bochdalek's hernia survive.

Cleft lip and palate

Cleft lip and cleft palate both have incidences of around 1/1000; when the anomalies are combined the incidence is 1.5/1000. Cleft lip may vary from a small dimple in the vermilion border to severe bilateral cleft.

The cleft palate may not be obvious at birth and is screened for on routine neonatal check by direct vision and palpation. There may be problems with feeding early on and it is important to involve the local orthodontist and speech therapist. Many regional centres have a cleft lip and palate team with an on-call service. These specialist teams perform all surgical repairs. The age at which repair is undertaken is variable; there is some suggestion that early repair gives better results, but many centres wait until 3–6 months of age when the child is larger.

Early on there may be feeding difficulties. Later problems with glue ear and speech production predominate, with problems of body image later in life.

Exomphalos and gastroschisis

Defects of the anterior abdominal wall, these have an incidence of 1/6000 births, with an equal sex ratio. Both are caused by a failure of the intestine to return to the abdominal cavity during early uterine development because of a a lack of closing of the embryological folds which make up the wall.

In exomphalos the intestine is contained in a sac; the liver, which may be abnormally lobulated, may also be present there. This condition is frequently accompanied by other congenital anomalies, such as cardiac defects and chromosomal anomalies.

Gastroschisis babies are frequently low birth weight and rarely have associated anomalies. The bowel is not contained in a sac and the infants rapidly lose fluid and heat. In general the outlook is good with 85% of cases being easily reduced back into the abdomen.

Antenatal diagnosis should be possible in both these conditions as maternal alpha fetoprotein levels are elevated, and large lesions may be visualized on scan from 14–16 weeks. By 18–20 weeks even smaller defects should be detected.

Tracheo-oesophageal fistula

This anomaly occurs in 1/2500–3000 births. Eighty-five per cent of these have a blind-ending oesophageal pouch, with a fistula from the trachea to the lower portion of the oesophagus; 10% have no fistula. An 'H' type fistula with no atresia rarely occurs.

The commonest type frequently presents with polyhydramnios alerting clinicians to swallowing problems. Other signs may include a baby who is constantly drooling or dribbling secretions or who chokes when offered feeds.

Passing a nasogastric tube and then X-raying for position may be diagnostic; 30–50% of babies may have associated anomalies such as radial problems, renal tract abnormalities and cardiac defects.

Overall the prognosis is good, the aim of surgery being to reconnect the oesophagus, and divide any fistulae. In babies over 1.5 kg the survival rate is around 95%.

Neural tube disorders

Neural tube disorders such as spina bifida, anencephaly and hydrocephalus have been diminishing in incidence over the last 30 years.

The reasons for this are not fully understood; it may partly be the result of antenatal diagnosis and termination of pregnancy in severe cases, but also due to vitamin supplementation of pregnant women with folic acid 4 mg daily from before conception to at least the 12th week of pregnancy. There are also other reasons, which are not entirely clear, and there are significant regional variations throughout the UK.

Antenatal diagnosis consists of monitoring serum alpha fetoprotein in pregnancy. This, however, is non-specific, as other abnormalities may give rise to high levels. Ultrasound scanning can detect lesions such as spina bifida and anencephaly (see p. 192). Risk of recurrence to siblings is around 5%.

Spina bifida

This is the name given to several lesions in which there is disruption of the vertebral arches. There may be a meningocele, in which there is a skin-covered lesion containing no neural tissue. Here the prognosis is good.

In the case of a myelomeningocele, where the neural plate is exposed, or covered by a thin layer of tissue, many infants die. Of those who survive, 90% will have hydrocephalus and severe orthopaedic problems.

Anencephaly

In this condition the skull bones fail to fuse and the brain is malformed with absent cerebral hemispheres. There may be other associated abnormalities such as spina bifida, and polyhydramnios is frequently present (see p. 185).

The condition is incompatible with survival, although some infants may live for a number of days; genetic couselling is important for parents due to the increased risk of neural tube anomalies in subsequent children.

Hydrocephalus

This may be congenital due to obstruction of CSF flow, most commonly occurring at the aqueduct of Sylvius. Rarely it may be because of over-production of CSF.

It may be acquired after birth as a complication of conditions such as neonatal meningitis or intraventricular haemorrhage.

Cranial ultrasound is easily performed when it is suspected, and it is commonly treated by insertion of a ventriculoperitoneal shunt.

Hydronephrosis

Frequently diagnosed on antenatal ultrasound, it is important to diagnose as this condition may be associated with reflux nephropathy leading to renal failure in later life.

Identified babies should be placed on antibiotic prophylaxis after birth and receive further ultrasound imaging according to local policy.

Ambiguous genitalia

This is a very difficult and distressing problem for parents and staff, and the parents must be told of the problem as soon as possible. No gender should be assigned to the baby until further investigation has taken place.

A careful examination of the infant should be undertaken, including the genitalia. Palpable gonads are usually testes and may be a vital clue.

Urgent investigations should be undertaken and must include chromosomal analysis, and measurement of 17-hydroxyprogesterone and electrolytes.

The commonest cause of ambiguous genitalia is congenital adrenal hyperplasia caused by 21-hydroxylase deficiency in the cortisol pathway. Virilization of a female fetus occurs and salt-wasting may occur due to lack of mineralocorticoid.

Hirschsprung's disease

This may present as late passage of meconium. Ninety-four per cent of babies will pass meconium in the first 24 hours of life and delay past this point should be taken seriously.

Abdominal distension and vomiting will be present but signs of obstruction are incomplete. This condition is caused by aganglionosis of the distal rectum. The sex preponderance is 4:1 males to females.

Diagnosis may be made on barium enema, but a definitive diagnosis requires rectal biopsy.

Treatment is by surgical resection of the affected portion with end to end anastomosis.

CHROMOSOMAL ABNORMALITIES

Down's syndrome

The commonest chromosomal abnormality, occurring as a result of trisomy 21, there is an incidence of 1/600 births, increasing with maternal age up to 1/100 at age 40.

Babies have typical facies with short palpebral fissures, up-slanting eyes, a large tongue and flat occiput. Hypotonia and poor feeding are common in infants. Forty per cent have cardiac lesions, usually endocardial cushion defects.

Patau syndrome

The result of trisomy 13, this occurs in 1/7000 births.

Most babies die in the first 12 months. Microcephaly is common, and 80% have heart defects.

Edwards' syndrome

Caused by trisomy 18, this occurs in 1/5000 births.

Most babies die in the first 12 months. Small stature is typical, with 'rocker-bottom' feet and cardiac and renal lesions.

CARDIAC ANOMALIES

The incidence is 0.8% of live births. Many present on routine examination, but some present as a collapsed, shocked, cyanosed baby, or with breathlessness and poor feeding.

Hypoplastic left-heart often presents early as a collapsed neonate; the prognosis is very poor, although operative treatments are available.

Many lesions such as coarctation of the aorta are duct-dependent and only present when the ductus arteriosus closes. This may occur in the first few days, but may not close for a number of weeks, leading to late presentation of some serious lesions. A soft transient systolic murmur is often heard in the first few days of life, caused by a closing patent ductus arteriosus.

Babies should be investigated with a chest X-ray, ECG and oxygen saturation measurement, whenever a cardiac lesion is suspected.

INFECTION

Chlamydia

This usually presents as conjunctivitis. Special swabs must be sent for analysis and treatment with oral erythromycin as well as topical therapy must be given.

Group B streptococcus

This is carried in the genital tract of around 25% of all women, and may cause a rapidly fatal illness in the neonatal period. This may present in a manner similar to respiratory distress syndrome, that is with grunting, tachypnoea and apnoea, or it may present with acute collapse and shock; 60% present in the first 24 hours. Even in treated neonates, mortality is 10%. If the mother is known to carry Group B Streptococcus, and has received antibiotics in labour, then the baby should receive 5 days penicillin and an aminoglycoside such as gentamicin.

A term baby who is otherwise healthy may be carefully observed on a post-natal ward without receiving antibiotics. Antibiotics will not eradicate carriage in the genital tract.

Herpes simplex
This may be a congenital infection leading to skin vesicles at birth, CNS lesions and eye involvement, often chorioretinitis.

Neurological handicap is common.

It is more commonly acquired at delivery from the genital tract, mainly HSV2.

Infection will occur in one-third of primary maternal cases, but is rare in reactivation.

Rubella
This is very rare since the introduction of MMR vaccine in 1988; fewer than 10 cases per year were recorded in a 10-year period.

Rubella can cause petechiae, microphthalmia, cataracts and hepatosplenomegaly.

Cytomegalovirus
The commonest congenital infection causing disease in the newborn, it may cause petechiae, hepatosplenomegaly, microcephaly, hearing loss, jaundice and intracranial calcification. The diagnostic test is viral culture from urine.

Prolonged rupture of membranes
Local policies vary, but if membranes are ruptured for more than 24 hours, the baby needs close observation of temperature, pulse and feeding, and any deterioration should be assumed to be infection and treated with appropriate broad-spectrum antibiotics, often benzylpenicillin or ampicillin, with an aminoglycoside.

An asymptotic term baby needs no therapy.

Varicella zoster
If contracted by the mother before 20 weeks' gestation this may rarely cause congenital infection, leading to growth retardation and convulsions, carrying a poor prognosis.

If the mother develops a chickenpox rash within 5 days of delivery then infection is severe with a high mortality. The infant should be treated with zoster immunoglobulin.

RESPIRATORY PROBLEMS

Transient tachypnoea of the newborn

This occurs in full-term babies and is caused by delayed clearance of fetal lung fluid. It is usually a mild illness presenting with tachypnoea, grunting, but with little or no requirement for supplementary oxygen – usually only 30–40%. It is usually resolves within 24–48 hours. It is common after Caesarean section.

Pneumothorax

There is a high incidence of 1% of all term babies although most are asymptomatic. It is commoner in babies with lung disease such as respiratory distress syndrome.

Symptoms include tachypnoea, restlessness, grunting and sudden collapse if the pneumothorax is under tension. Small lesions may require no treatment, however where symptoms are more severe a chest drain will need to be inserted.

Pneumonia

This may be difficult to distinguish from other forms of respiratory distress. The most serious form is caused by Group B Streptococcus, but it may also be caused by *E. coli*, Listeria, and *Staphylococcus aureus*.

METABOLIC DISORDERS

Many of these conditions exist and most are individually rare. They are important because they are part of the differential diagnosis of a collapsed newborn, along with infections and severe cardiac lesion. These are more common in families where there is consanguinity, a history of unexplained neonatal deaths, or undiagnosed neurological illness in a sibling.

NEUROLOGICAL PROBLEMS

Hypoxic ischaemic encephalopathy

This is the correct term for 'birth asphyxia'. It consists of alterations in level of consciousness, seizures, altered muscle tone and behaviour, and may be categorized into three stages:

Stage 1 describes mild disease, hyper-alertness and normal muscle tone, which is short lived.

Stage 2 seizures are common, with mild hypotonia, lasting 2–14 days.

Stage 3 describes severe disease: the babies are stuporose, flaccid and may be apnoeic, this period lasting hours to weeks.

Outcome varies according to stage. All stage 1 and many stage 2 babies will have normal neurological outcomes. At stage 3, 60% will die and most survivors have significant handicap.

Seizures

These are not uncommon in the neonatal period. They are usually the result of a pathological process, although some may be benign.

The commonest cause is hypoxic ischaemic encephalopathy, other causes being intracranial haemorrhage from birth trauma, CNS infections and metabolic derangement, such as hypoglycaemia, hypocalcaemia or inborn errors of metabolism.

Familial neonatal seizures occur as an autosomal dominant phenomenon, also benign neonatal sleep myoclonus.

Babies presenting with seizures should undergo careful examination, and should be investigated for infection. Electrolytes, calcium, glucose and magnesium must be checked in the first instance.

RESUSCITATION

The Royal College of Paediatrics and Child Health and the Royal College of Obstetricians and Gynaecologists have produced national guidelines (see Figs 7.1 and 7.2).

It is recommended that at each delivery there is one dedicated person looking after the baby who has been trained in neonatal resuscitation.

Most term babies do not require resuscitation, facial oxygen or nasopharyngeal suction; merely to be dried and wrapped in a warm dry towel!

Resuscitation Chart 1

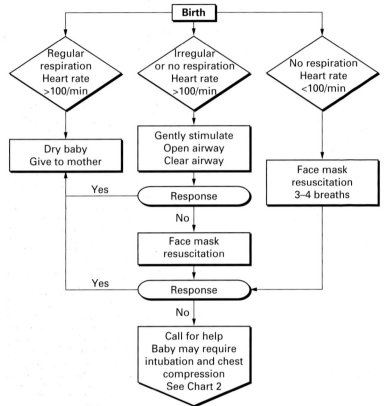

Fig. 7.1 Current national guidelines for resuscitation. Resuscitation charts 1 and 2, reproduced from Royal College of Paediatrics and Child Health and Royal College of Obstetricians and Gynaecologists, *Resuscitation of Babies at Birth*. BMJ 1997.

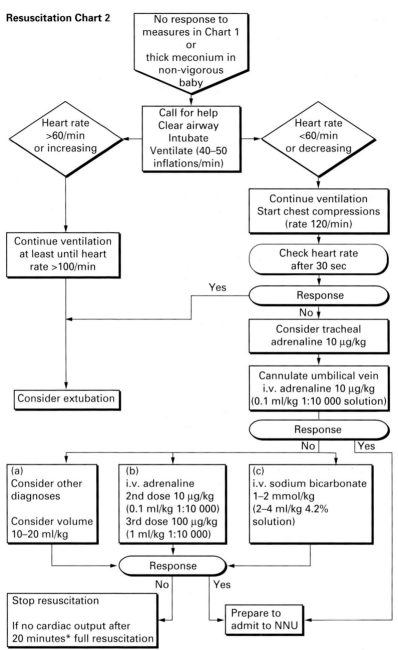

Resuscitation Chart 2

No response to measures in Chart 1 or thick meconium in non-vigorous baby

Call for help
Clear airway
Intubate
Ventilate (40–50 inflations/min)

Heart rate >60/min or increasing

Heart rate <60/min or decreasing

Continue ventilation at least until heart rate >100/min

Continue ventilation
Start chest compressions (rate 120/min)

Check heart rate after 30 sec

Response — Yes

No

Consider tracheal adrenaline 10 µg/kg

Cannulate umbilical vein
i.v. adrenaline 10 µg/kg
(0.1 ml/kg 1:10 000 solution)

Consider extubation

Response

No   Yes

(a)
Consider other diagnoses

Consider volume 10–20 ml/kg

(b)
i.v. adrenaline
2nd dose 10 µg/kg
(0.1 ml/kg 1:10 000)
3rd dose 100 µg/kg
(1 ml/kg 1:10 000)

(c)
i.v. sodium bicarbonate
1–2 mmol/kg
(2–4 ml/kg 4.2% solution)

Response

No   Yes

Stop resuscitation

If no cardiac output after 20 minutes* full resuscitation

Prepare to admit to NNU

(a) Consider whilst preparing for (b) ± (c) depending on local policy.
*May vary with individual circumstances and local guidelines.
i.v. = intravenous; NNU = neonatal unit.

Fig. 7.2

APPENDIX

Royal College of Obstetricians and Gynaecologists

27 SUSSEX PLACE, REGENT'S PARK, LONDON NW1 4RG
Telephone: +44 (0)207-772 6200

Diploma Examination (DRCOG)
Detailed Instructions for the
Multiple Choice Question Paper
in Obstetrics and Gynaecology

This information must be read very carefully. Failure to follow the instructions will result in failure in the examination.

IDENTIFICATION
Candidates must provide evidence of identification, **which includes name and photograph,** for inspection prior to commencement of the examination. Candidates failing to provide satisfactory evidence will not be allowed to attend the examination.

REGISTRATION FOR THE EXAMINATION
The MCQ Paper will be held in the morning **or** afternoon depending on the session that you have been allocated. Candidates sitting the MCQ Paper in the morning will attend the OSCE in the afternoon. Those candidates allocated the OSCE in the morning will attend the MCQ Paper in the afternoon. You must register for the morning session (MCQ Paper or OSCE) by the time stated on your entry card. **Candidates failing to register on time will be withdrawn from the examination.**

THE QUESTION PAPER
The paper will consist of sixty (5 part) Multiple Choice Questions in book form. A computer Answer Sheet on which answers are to be recorded will be inserted into the Question Book and this sheet will be marked by a document reading machine. A sample computer Answer Sheet is shown overleaf. **You must use only the grade HB pencil provided for completing all parts of the Answer Sheet.** Pens must not be used for any part of the MCQ examination. Firm pressure is required with the pencil. You must ensure that your marking is bold and dark. You may erase any pencil mark by using the eraser provided. The time allowed for completion of the MCQ examination is TWO hours. You will be given a time warning 30 minutes and 10 minutes before the end of the examination. **Do not start the examination until instructed by the invigilator.**

FRONT COVER
On the front cover of the Question Book you must print your full name in the boxes provided and then sign your name in the space marked "signature". Your candidate number (not desk number) must be written in the FOUR SQUARES labelled "CANDIDATE NUMBER".

ANSWER SHEET (Sample overleaf)
A FIRM DARK IMPRESSION WHICH COMPLETELY FILLS EACH LOZENGE IS ESSENTIAL.

A FAINT LINE WILL NOT BE READ BY THE DOCUMENT READING MACHINE.

The Answer Sheet must not be folded, creased or torn. You must print your surname (family name) and other name(s) at the top of the Answer Sheet and write your <u>CANDIDATE</u> <u>NUMBER</u> in the boxes provided. Then **black-out** the lozenges corresponding to your candidate number.

YOU MUST SHOW YOUR NAME AS STATED ON YOUR ENTRY CARD.

QUESTIONS

Each question will consist of an initial statement followed by five items identified by the letters A, B, C, D, E. The answer sheet contains a row of five boxes for each question and is numbered accordingly. Each box refers to a single item. In each box there are two lozenges labelled T(= True) and F(= False). You will be required to indicate whether you know a particular item to be true or false by **boldly** blacking out either the True or False lozenge.

To avoid too many erasures on the answer sheet, candidates may wish to mark their responses in the Question Book and then transfer their decisions to the Answer Sheet but this **must** be done **within** the two hours allowed for the examination.

Specimen question and answers

There is a recognised association between polyhydramnios and
A. twin pregnancy
B. fetal abnormality
C. fetal growth retardation
D. cord prolapse
E. post partum haemorrhage

Answers A, B, D and E are 'True', answer C is 'False'. Your answer sheet relating to this question would look like this when correctly filled in:

A   B   C   D   E

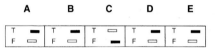

T means TRUE: F means FALSE

MARKING

Each item correctly answered (i.e. a True statement indicated as True or a False statement indicated as False) is awarded one mark (+1). For each incorrect answer no mark (0) is awarded. **All items must be answered true or false. Incorrect answers are not penalised.**

COMPLETION

At the end of the examination insert the completed Answer Sheet into the Question Book.

On no account may the Question Book be removed from the examination hall.

Any candidate who attempts to remove, by writing or by any other means, MCQ examination questions from the examination hall, will be reported to the Examination Committee and will FAIL the whole examination.

Royal College of Obstetricians and Gynaecologists
Diploma Examination (DRCOG)

SURNAME (FAMILY NAME) JOHNSON

OTHER NAME(S) PETER ALAN

Please use HB pencil. Rub out all errors thoroughly.
Mark lozenges like ▬ NOT like ✓ X O

T = True
F = False

CANDIDATE NUMBER

1 2 7 5

IMPORTANT NOTES

1. When you have finished, check that you have NOT left any blanks.

2. Erasures should be left clean, with no smudges where possible. (The document reading machine will accept the darkest response for each item).

	A	B	C	D	E
1	T / F	T / F	T / F	T / F	T / F
2	T / F	T / F	T / F	T / F	T / F
3	T / F	T / F	T / F	T / F	T / F
4	T / F	T / F	T / F	T / F	T / F
5	T / F	T / F	T / F	T / F	T / F
6	T / F	T / F	T / F	T / F	T / F
7	T / F	T / F	T / F	T / F	T / F
8	T / F	T / F	T / F	T / F	T / F
9	T / F	T / F	T / F	T / F	T / F
10	T / F	T / F	T / F	T / F	T / F
11	T / F	T / F	T / F	T / F	T / F
12	T / F	T / F	T / F	T / F	T / F
13	T / F	T / F	T / F	T / F	T / F
14	T / F	T / F	T / F	T / F	T / F
15	T / F	T / F	T / F	T / F	T / F

	A	B	C	D	E
16	T / F	T / F	T / F	T / F	T / F
17	T / F	T / F	T / F	T / F	T / F
18	T / F	T / F	T / F	T / F	T / F
19	T / F	T / F	T / F	T / F	T / F
20	T / F	T / F	T / F	T / F	T / F
21	T / F	T / F	T / F	T / F	T / F
22	T / F	T / F	T / F	T / F	T / F
23	T / F	T / F	T / F	T / F	T / F
24	T / F	T / F	T / F	T / F	T / F
25	T / F	T / F	T / F	T / F	T / F
26	T / F	T / F	T / F	T / F	T / F
27	T / F	T / F	T / F	T / F	T / F
28	T / F	T / F	T / F	T / F	T / F
29	T / F	T / F	T / F	T / F	T / F
30	T / F	T / F	T / F	T / F	T / F

CHECK THAT YOU HAVE ANSWERED EVERY ITEM TRUE OR FALSE

Please use HB pencil. Rub out all errors thoroughly.
Mark lozenges like ▬ NOT like ✓ ✗ ○

T = True
F = False

IMPORTANT NOTES

1. When you have finished, check that you have NOT left any blanks.
2. Erasures should be left clean, with no smudges where possible. (The document reading machine will accept the darkest response for each item).

	A	B	C	D	E		A	B	C	D	E
31	T F	T F	T F	T F	T F	**46**	T F	T F	T F	T F	T F
32	T F	T F	T F	T F	T F	**47**	T F	T F	T F	T F	T F
33	T F	T F	T F	T F	T F	**48**	T F	T F	T F	T F	T F
34	T F	T F	T F	T F	T F	**49**	T F	T F	T F	T F	T F
35	T F	T F	T F	T F	T F	**50**	T F	T F	T F	T F	T F
36	T F	T F	T F	T F	T F	**51**	T F	T F	T F	T F	T F
37	T F	T F	T F	T F	T F	**52**	T F	T F	T F	T F	T F
38	T F	T F	T F	T F	T F	**53**	T F	T F	T F	T F	T F
39	T F	T F	T F	T F	T F	**54**	T F	T F	T F	T F	T F
40	T F	T F	T F	T F	T F	**55**	T F	T F	T F	T F	T F
41	T F	T F	T F	T F	T F	**56**	T F	T F	T F	T F	T F
42	T F	T F	T F	T F	T F	**57**	T F	T F	T F	T F	T F
43	T F	T F	T F	T F	T F	**58**	T F	T F	T F	T F	T F
44	T F	T F	T F	T F	T F	**59**	T F	T F	T F	T F	T F
45	T F	T F	T F	T F	T F	**60**	T F	T F	T F	T F	T F

CHECK THAT YOU HAVE ANSWERED EVERY ITEM TRUE OR FALSE

INDEX